Nursing and Informatics for the 21st Century – Embracing a Digital World, 3rd Edition, Book 1

Nursing and Informatics for the 21st Century – Embracing a Digital World, 3rd Edition is comprised of four books which can be purchased individually at www.routledge.com:

Book 1: Realizing Digital Health – Bold Challenges and Opportunities for Nursing – ISBN: 9780367516888

Book 2: Nursing Education and Digital Health Strategies – ISBN: 9781032249728

Book 3: Innovation, Technology, and Applied Informatics for Nurses – ISBN: 9781032249803

Book 4: Nursing in an Integrated Digital World that Supports People, Systems, and the Planet – ISBN: 9781032249827

Nursing and Informatics for the 21st Century – Embracing a Digital World, 3rd Edition, Book 1

Realizing Digital Health – Bold Challenges and Opportunities for Nursing

Edited by

Connie White Delaney, PhD, RN, FAAN, FACMI, FNAP
Charlotte A. Weaver, PhD, MSPH, RN, FHIMSS, FAAN
Joyce Sensmeier, MS, RN-BC, FHIMSS, FAAN
Lisiane Pruinelli, PhD, MS, RN, FAMIA
Patrick Weber, MA, RN, FIAHSI, FGBHI

Foreword by Deborah Trautman, PhD, RN, FAAN
President and Chief Executive Officer,
American Association of Colleges of Nursing

Foreword by Kedar Mate, MD
President and CEO,
Institute for Healthcare Improvement

Foreword by Howard Catton
Chief Executive Officer,
International Council of Nurses

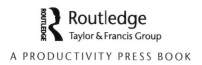

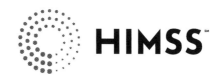

A PRODUCTIVITY PRESS BOOK

First published 2022
by Routledge
605 Third Avenue, New York, NY 10158

and by Routledge
2 Park Square, Milton Park, Abingdon, Oxon, OX14 4RN

Routledge is an imprint of the Taylor & Francis Group, an informa business

ISBN: 9780367516895 (hbk)
ISBN: 9780367516888 (pbk)
ISBN: 9781003054849 (ebk)

DOI: 10.4324/9781003054849

Typeset in Garamond
by Deanta Global Publishing Services, Chennai, India

Dedication for Connie White Delaney

Responding to the urgent and powerful invitation for community, partnership and collaboration, this *Nursing and Informatics for the 21st Century—Embracing a Digital World*, 3rd Edition is dedicated to all individuals, organizations and informaticians who are co-creating futures, health and healthcare. May these co-created informatics-anchored futures radiate the brain of intellect and wisdom, the brain of heart and compassion, and the action brain of impact, voice, caring and awakening.

Dedication for Charlotte A. Weaver

Reflecting these painful times, this dedication goes out to all our frontline nurses and fellow healthcare workers who have taken care of us all around the globe at the risk of their own lives and well-being. We owe you.

Dedication for Joyce Sensmeier

To my husband and life partner who has faithfully supported my informatics journey, encouraging me to take risks along the way, and congratulating me on every success. Thank you for believing in me.

Dedication for Lisiane Pruinelli

To those who battle every day for a better world … 'I don't write a book so that it will be the final word; I write a book so that other books are possible, not necessarily written by me.' —Michel Foucault

Dedication for Patrick Weber

For the sake of the population, the empowerment of nurses worldwide is the best effort to improve disease prevention and promote good health. Thank you to my co-editors and all the authors for their work on this book series.

Contents

Foreword

When the nation's nursing school deans voted to endorse *The Essentials: Core Competencies for Professional Nursing Education* in April 2021, new competency expectations for tomorrow's nurses came into focus. Driven in part by the need to ensure consistency among graduates of entry-level and advanced-level nursing education programs, one area receiving special emphasis across roles is nursing informatics. As we considered how best to prepare professional nurses to thrive in the future, the need for providers to 'use information and communication technologies and informatics processes to deliver safe nursing care to diverse populations in a variety of settings' (Essential 8.3) was affirmed as a key competency expectation.

Over the past 20 years, informatics increasingly has been a focus in nursing education, given the rapid rise in the use of technology to guide healthcare delivery and clinical decision-making and the need to critically consider all available data when engaging in evidence-based practice and precision healthcare. Basic informatics competencies are foundational to all nursing practice.

Reaching this point in the evolution of our understanding of informatics would not have been possible without pioneers in the field. The authors of *Nursing and Informatics for the 21st Century—Embracing a Digital World*, 3rd Edition—Connie White Delaney, Charlotte A. Weaver, Joyce Sensmeier, Lisiane Pruinelli and Patrick Weber—stand among the world's leading authorities on health informatics, data science and digital health. Committed to enhancing the scholarship of discovery, these nurse leaders are known internationally for their trailblazing work that has been recognized by such authorities as the Alliance for Nursing Informatics, American Medical Informatics Association, International Academy of Health Sciences Informatics and the Healthcare Information and Management Systems Society. Their pedigrees are undeniable, their thought leadership profound.

The publication of this expansive resource comes at a time when nursing is once again divining its future into the next decade. In addition to the re-envisioned AACN's *Essentials*, which is setting a new standard for nursing education, recent National Academy of Medicine reports on *The Future of Nursing* and *Implementing High Quality Primary Care* point the way forward for nursing practice, research priorities and interprofessional engagement. All these paths demand a greater understanding and reliance on informatics as a driver of innovation and impact. Further, healthcare's move to address pressing social needs, including a shared desire to achieve health equity, gain insight into the social determinants of health, expand consumer access to data and attend to global health concerns are all considered within the context of digital technologies and applied data science as part of this new book series.

Nursing and Informatics for the 21st Century—Embracing a Digital World, 3rd Edition will be of great interest to nurses and other health professionals in the US and globally who are eager to learn more about leveraging automated systems and emerging science to sustain health and improve healthcare delivery. This book series serves as an important resource for practice leaders, nurse researchers, systems analysts, healthcare consumers and graduate students looking to explore opportunities for innovation that develop at the nexus of nursing science, emerging technologies, critical thinking and patient-centered care.

As we look to a future with nursing education that is more competency-based, informatics will be front and center. For faculty wishing to keep pace with the latest thinking on contemporary nursing education and practice, this essential resource will help to inform your understanding about the value and reach of informatics and may also generate new ideas for developing experiential learning opportunities using artificial intelligence, telehealth, simulation and other leading-edge technologies. These emerging tools and practices are transforming nursing roles as well as the skills and knowledge needed to manage care remotely. This comprehensive work will help lead conversations to inspire future generations of nurses to explore how best to leverage nursing informatics in their research, practice and leadership roles.

Deborah Trautman, PhD, RN, FAAN
President and Chief Executive Officer
American Association of Colleges of Nursing

Foreword

Walk onto any clinical service unit in a modern hospital, and you will realize that clinical practice today is a fully socio-technological phenomenon—entirely reliant both upon a nurse's compassion and upon our technology's capacity to supply information and services just in time. Technologies are no longer working their way into health and healthcare—they are already integral to both. But the promise of these incredibly exciting digital therapeutics, diagnostics and monitoring systems depends on, just as more conventional medicines have for decades, the human systems required to implement them. This interface—between nurses and the digital information that can make care more effective, efficient, and reliable—is at the heart of 21st-century nursing informatics.

Years ago, the field of quality improvement in healthcare started with a simple premise—we could work on those human processes to take the fruits of clinical science—medications, new diagnostic assays, vaccines—and more reliably deliver them to patients to create lasting health effects. It is time for a complementary agenda—quality and reliability sciences must now be applied to improve the delivery of proven digital therapies and diagnostics. Just as we created reliable workflows that delivered antibiotics that would prevent sepsis deaths, so too must we create workflows that will leverage new data sources and technologies to improve the way we care for patients. Digital will change healthcare just as antibiotics have, but neither will achieve impact without implementation methods that ensure that the 'medicine' gets to the patient.

This is crucial because of the incredible potential of technology and data to improve care and outcomes. Consider how good artificial intelligence (AI)-guided diagnosis and triage have become: for some clinical conditions, AI now gets diagnostic and treatment accuracy over 90% right compared to clinicians in urgent care environments. These technologies won't replace the nurse or the physician, but they can radically affect the capacity of a clinician to see patients. If much of the time-consuming fact-finding, differential diagnosis, care plan documentation, and charting can be done by an AI-guided automated assistant, nurses can spend much more time caring for patients.

Realizing technology's transformative potential in nursing requires a comprehensive understanding of how to turn data into information; information into knowledge; knowledge into wisdom; and wisdom into applied practice. This book series is essential to such an understanding. This new edition is a detailed and exhaustive exploration of the myriad contexts, approaches, challenges and success stories of how effective informatics can improve every dimension of health, including the fiercely urgent dimensions of needing to improve access to care and ensuring health equity.

For those new to the field of informatics, this series contains an illuminating history of the rapid and profound changes in digital health over the past decade. And for those with deep experience in the field, there are chapters detailing both what's happening at the cutting-edge and what the future holds. Anyone who wants to improve nursing practice in the modern era needs to read this book series and heed its calls to action.

Kedar Mate, MD
President and CEO
Institute for Healthcare Improvement

Foreword

As the COVID-19 pandemic has so painfully shown us, it is hard to accurately predict the future. While the temptation is to spend time and effort on futurology—it can be hard to resist—our time is probably better spent on trying to prepare flexibly for what is coming next and, in some way, help to shape it.

What seems certain is that digital health will feature in our futures and that nurses are in a prime position to take advantage of the benefits it can bring. In fact, as we have seen, recent developments in digital health are some of the few positives to have come out of the pandemic.

Finding ways to deal with the pandemic brought about a rapid increase in access to digitally enhanced care, whether it be through the use of video-conferencing for consultations and telehealth or through increased access to massive amounts of data that were previously buried and heavily guarded in the depths of healthcare organizations' information technology systems. The issue now is understanding the data and using it meaningfully to improve services and reduce costs.

While only a year or so ago it would have been correct to say the future is digital, we can now say that, in many parts of the world, digital health is already here and that it looks like it's here to stay. We can see it in the development of nurse-led models of care and how the use of data and new equipment is changing the traditional, paternalistic models of care to more responsive ones that are personalized, faster, sustainable and more affordable.

The biggest challenge ahead will be to expand access to nursing informatics to all nurses, wherever they are so that they can provide equitable access to state-of-the-art care to people everywhere.

This is especially important as the world deals with and recovers from the COVID-19 pandemic. Nurse-led models of care, underpinned by access to data, are a big part of the solution as we strengthen our health systems for the post-pandemic world to come.

I am delighted to write this foreword for what is likely to be a very influential book series about nursing and informatics and how nurses can maximize the impact of digital health for the benefit of patients and their families and the health systems that they work in.

In the past, information technology has promised so much but often failed to deliver on its potential. If it is to fulfil its promise, it must be an enabler for people to be empowered, and it must improve access to services, the quality and efficiency of those services, and the patient's care and health outcomes.

For this to happen, the people on the receiving end of care need to be at the centre of the systems that are developed, and nurses must be involved in all stages of their design, development and implementation. In the past, we have seen how the ill-thought-out introduction of some systems has taken nurses away from direct care, to the detriment of their patients and the annoyance of the nurses.

Nurses do not want to spend hours in front of computer screens, as they have been required to in the past. They do not want to spend their time inputting data into counterintuitive systems that do not meet their requirements. What they want is quick and easy access to the information they need at their fingertips, in people's homes, at the nurses' station on wards, at the bedside and in the clinics where they work, in real time while they are interacting with their patients.

We see the power of technology and data-driven change across the globe, from low- to high-income settings, from the use of Apps on mobile phones to the adoption of sophisticated information systems and algorithms. But underlying it all is the continuing need for a highly skilled and educated nursing workforce. Whatever the future holds in terms of information technology, artificial intelligence and robotics, they will always be used in support of the compassion, the relationships and the dynamic human factors that only nurses can provide.

This *Nursing and Informatics for the 21st Century—Embracing a Digital World*, 3rd Edition shows the path ahead for our profession to become fully digitally enabled. I am sure it will prove to be an indispensable guide along the way.

Howard Catton
Chief Executive Officer
International Council of Nurses

Preface

While we commit to living in the 21st century and maintaining our open minds and hearts to the needs, wishes and wisdom that will inform our future, we have found the pace of change to be challenging in preparing this book series. Every day, new technologies and partnerships are in the social news media, and healthcare systems announce new digital health programs that push care out into the hands of patients and into the home. Additionally, these new care modalities and technology changes are occurring simultaneously with national and international policy mandates to address social injustices and inequities, equality in access to care, and planetary health. Tremendous innovation has transpired since the publication of this book's second edition in 2010. In that space of time, medical sensing devices and mobile technologies have become ubiquitous, permeating every aspect of our lives. Concurrently, the synergistic effect of new technologies and tools such as cloud data storage, application programming interfaces, artificial intelligence and machine learning are game changers in advancing digital health. Together with legislation and regulatory changes, the proprietary limitations of electronic health record (EHR) systems have been upended. The voice of the consumer and insistence on patient-centered, connected and readily accessible care have never had greater velocity, urging our unremitting attention.

Thus, in planning this third edition, we abandoned the previous framework of presenting an 'international snapshot of current state' on EHR adoption and nursing. Technology changes and new applications that extract data, apply AI systems, dashboards, and suggest care protocols made a primary EHR framework irrelevant. Increasingly, economics and policy mandates push healthcare systems to embrace a preventative, wellness and population health focus that requires new thinking toward advanced technology applications that extend services into clinics, community and the home. In the United States, reimbursement linked to Alternative Payment Models (APM) and 'value-based purchasing' with dependency on quality metrics require healthcare systems to collaborate with community resources and post-acute care providers. All collaboration, local to world-wide, demands exchanging and sharing information, as well as actively engaging individual patients and their families. A plethora of digital/mobile applications have emerged to fill this evolving 'non-acute care/non-EHR' space. As chapters from geographic areas spanning the globe describe, economic imperatives, mandates to deliver equal access to care in rural as well as metro areas, and the need to incorporate social determinants of health into care delivery have also driven the adoption of digital health solutions. Therefore, this third edition focuses on these new technologies and the care delivery models they make possible: thus, we gave this work the subtitle *'Embracing a Digital World.'*

Kristine Mednansky, Senior Editor from Taylor & Francis Group, LLC, asked us to consider a new edition, based on feedback from the readers of our previous works. Our full gratitude goes to Ms Mednansky for this series' existence. Her voice was the key driver for creating this work, the *Nursing and Informatics for the 21st Century*, 3rd Edition. Ms Mednansky ensured that this current work would meet the needs of readers in a variety of formats: electronic, print, and the option to purchase either an individual chapter or an entire book. Moreover, readers will note another major difference in the look and feel of the previous hardcover book: this work has been converted to a four-book series to deliver a resource that is more easily consumed. Our hope is that with this flexibility in access and usability, the work embodied in this collection of contributing authors will be widely read and extensively shared. We look forward to receiving your feedback on this novel approach.

This work is organized into a series of four books, each with 11 chapters: (1) Realizing Digital Health–Bold Challenges and Opportunities for Nursing; (2) Nursing Education and Digital Health Strategies; (3) Innovation, Technology, and Applied Informatics for Nurses; and (4) Nursing in an Integrated Digital World that Supports People, Systems, and the Planet. Each book in the series includes international contributors with authors from Africa and South Africa, Brazil, Belgium, Canada, China, England, Finland, Germany, Italy, Norway, the Philippines, South Korea, Sri Lanka, Switzerland, Taiwan, and the United States, as well as authors of additional exemplars from China, India and the West Balkan countries. Throughout this series, the wisdom of leading-edge innovators is interwoven with digital health applications, global thought leaders and multinational, cooperative research initiatives, all against the backdrop of health equity and policy-setting bodies, such as the United Nations and the World Health Organization.

We begin Book 1 of the series by introducing the paradigm of digital health, and its underlying technologies, offering examples of its potential use and future impacts. This introduction is followed by an in-depth look at the ethical considerations in digital health that nurses and informaticists need to understand, authored by an international team of nursing informatics leaders from Finland, Canada and England. The growing movement in consumerism and patient engagement is described in a collaborative research initiative between academia–government–industry. This chapter is bolstered by numerous exemplars, all illustrating the importance of the engaged patient enabled by new digital technologies with the goal of making possible comprehensive access to individuals' digital health information, regardless of system or location. Several chapters focus on the underlying need for terminology and data standards to capture the data necessary to enable new science and knowledge discoveries. Subsequent chapters outline the critical and urgent role that nurse executive leaders' play in advancing digital health, as well as the knowledge and skills needed to take advantage of new digital technologies. We follow with chapters on the role(s) of nursing informatics leaders in large, US health systems, as well as a global perspective from Brazil, Italy and the Philippines. To provide a clear understanding of the challenges facing the United Nations and World Health Organizations' goals for health equity and equality, we include a critical examination of South Africa's healthcare delivery system, technologies and nursing's role across these structural segments. We close Book 1 with a look at the information sharing needed to support true team care spanning multiple settings and systems.

Book 2 is dedicated to a deep examination of nursing education's best practices, strategies, and informatics competencies. The chapters included in Book 2 span nursing education and learning for applied critical thinking, including the use of technology, content, skills versus tools, the use of 'smart' systems for care delivery and the role of critical thinking as essential to nursing care delivery. These concepts are understood as a paradigm shift that must be incorporated into nursing and healthcare education. Best practices for workforce and degree-level education are presented in a description of Emory's Academic/Practice partnership focusing on disruption through nurse innovation enabled by all nurses and students having access to big data. This book closes with a review of innovative methodologies being used in simulation labs across the globe, including some uses of virtual and augmented reality simulations.

Book 3 defines the foundations of artificial intelligence (AI), machine learning (ML) and various digital technologies, including social media, the Internet of Things, telehealth and applied data analytics, all with a look toward the future state. The Applied Healthcare Data Science Roadmap is presented as a framework aiming to educate healthcare leaders on the use of data science principles and tools to inform decision-making. We focus particular attention on the cautions, potential for harm, and biases that artificial intelligence technologies and machine learning may pose in healthcare, with the role of advocate and protector from harm falling under the nurse's role. Book 3 concludes by outlining four case studies featuring innovations developed by nurses in response to COVID-19, which highlight the creative use of technologies to support patients, care providers and healthcare systems during the global pandemic.

We continue with a focus on the theme of enabling digital technologies in Book 4 as they are used to address planetary health issues and care equity across developing countries. Throughout the development of this series, the world has struggled with the core issues of equity in access to care, needed medical equipment and supplies and vaccines. Sustainability and global health policy are linked to the new digital technologies in the chapters that illustrate healthcare delivery modalities, which nurse innovators are developing, leading and using to deliver care to hard-to-reach populations for better population health. Social media use in South Korea for health messaging, community initiatives and nursing research are presented with additional references to other Asian countries. A US description of consumer engagement with patient ownership of all their medical records data is presented with the underlying technologies explained in simple, understandable terms. Additionally, we tapped experts to highlight the legal statutes, government regulations and civil rights law in place for patients' rights, privacy and confidentiality, and consents for the United States, the United Kingdom and the European Union. The next chapter in Book 4 is written by two participants of the 'Future of Nursing 2020–2030' task force who deliver an optimistic message. These authors recognize the work that needs to be done around health equity and equality and review nursing's role responsibilities to effect these changes. Their optimism comes from all the opportunities that social policy and enabling digital technologies make possible for nursing. The authors outline how these changes in care delivery models, the patient/provider role and dependence on digital tools all present opportunities for new nursing roles, access to expansive data resources for research with the exponential growth of our science base and for entrepreneurship.

We conclude this book series with a chapter written by the editors in which we envision the near future. We explore the impact that digital technologies will have on: a) how care is delivered, including expanding care settings into community and home; b) virtual monitoring; and c) the type and quantity of patient-generated data and how it is used to advance knowledge and care excellence. Ultimately these changes highlight the numerous ways that nursing roles and skill sets related to digital health are needed to support the global goal of equal access to health and care. We emphasize the necessity for partnering. We send the message that nursing, along with our transdisciplinary partners, is being called to lead and create unparalleled transformation of healthcare to person-centered, connected and accessible care anchored in digital health.

Acknowledgement

We share our deep gratitude with all of the persons, including care providers, researchers, educators, business and corporate leaders, and informatics experts in all settings, for requesting an update to the second edition of *Nursing and Informatics for the 21st Century*. Together, you recognized the value and synergy of nursing and informatics, the core function of informatics in shaping nursing, health and healthcare, and the reciprocal learning that a global perspective offers us. Thank you to Taylor & Francis Group, LLC, and especially Kristine Mednansky, Senior Editor, for giving us the opportunity to produce this third edition as a totally new body of work in this post-EHR era. But most especially, for your creativity and flexibility as we presented a book double our original plan. Thus, this third edition is presented as a four-book series enveloping *Nursing and Informatics for the 21st Century*. We are deeply humbled by the dedication, work and creativity of our contributing authors, many of whom formed teams that expanded across continents to be able to capture the fullest coverage and latest information. The contributors bring state-of-the-art knowledge, coupled with real-world practice and education. It is the integration of nursing and informatics knowledge and practice that will sustain our health, communities and planet. Last, we would be remiss not to say a deep thank you to Midori V. Green, our project manager par excellence, who kept us organized and on track through her diplomacy and hard work and without which we would not have made our deadlines.

In gratitude,

Connie White Delaney
Charlotte A. Weaver
Joyce Sensmeier
Lisiane Pruinelli
Patrick Weber

Editors

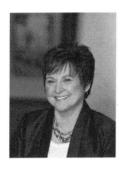

Connie White Delaney, PhD, RN, FAAN, FACMI, FNAP serves as Professor and Dean at the University of Minnesota School of Nursing and is the Knowledge Generation Lead for the National Center for Interprofessional Practice and Education. She served as Associate Director of the Clinical Translational Science Institute—Biomedical Informatics, and Acting Director of the Institute for Health Informatics (IHI) in the Academic Health Center from 2010 to 2015. She serves as an adjunct professor in the Faculty of Medicine and Faculty of Nursing at the University of Iceland, where she received the Doctor Scientiae Curationis Honoris Causa (Honorary Doctor of Philosophy in Nursing) in 2011. She is an elected Fellow in the American Academy of Nursing, American College of Medical Informatics, and National Academies of Practice. Delaney is the first Fellow in the College of Medical Informatics to serve as a Dean of Nursing. Delaney was an inaugural appointee to the USA Health Information Technology Policy Committee, Office of the National Coordinator, and Office of the Secretary for the U.S. Department of Health and Human Services (HHS). She is an active researcher in data and information technology standards for nursing, healthcare. Delaney is past president of Friends of the National Institute of Nursing Research (FNINR) and currently serves as Vice-Chair of CGFNS, Inc. She holds a BSN with majors in nursing and mathematics, MA in Nursing, PhD Educational Administration and Computer Applications, postdoctoral study in Nursing & Medical Informatics and a Certificate in Integrative Therapies & Healing Practices.

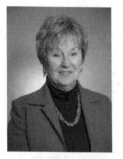

Charlotte A. Weaver, Ph.D., MSPH, RN, FHIMSS, FAAN is a visionary senior executive, now retired after 40+ years of experience in nursing informatics, patient safety and quality, evidence-based nursing practices and healthcare automation in acute, ambulatory and post-acute care. She created a breakthrough in the nursing educational curricula by introducing learning using an electronic health record (EHR) in virtual environments and pioneered the corporate-level, Chief Nurse Officer role. She also has Board Director experience in the public/non-profit healthcare sectors. With 15+ years of experience at the chief executive level in the corporate HIT industry and healthcare delivery organizations with Board-reporting responsibilities, her fields of specialization include EHR, health IT policy, post-acute care delivery in home health and hospice provider organizations. Dr. Weaver serves on a number of academic, healthcare systems and healthcare technology company Boards. She is a fellow in the American Academy of Nursing and the Health Information Management Systems Society (HIMSS). She is a frequent presenter at national and international conferences and has published extensively as a writer and editor. Dr. Weaver has a PhD in Medical Anthropology from the University of California, Berkeley and San Francisco, an MSPH in Epidemiology and a BA in Anthropology from the University of Washington, and a Nursing diploma from St Elizabeth's School of Nursing. She was a post-doctoral fellow at the University of Hawaii.

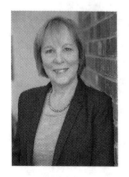

Joyce Sensmeier, MS, RN-BC, FHIMSS, FAAN is the Senior Advisor, Informatics for HIMSS, a non-profit organization focused on reforming the global health ecosystem through the power of information and technology. In this role, she provides thought leadership in the areas of clinical informatics, interoperability and standards programs and initiatives. Sensmeier served as Vice President, Informatics at HIMSS from 2005 to 2019. She is president of IHE USA, a non-profit organization whose mission is to improve our nation's healthcare by promoting the adoption and use of IHE and other world-class standards, tools and services for interoperability. An internationally recognized speaker and author of numerous book chapters and articles, Sensmeier achieved fellowship in the American Academy of Nursing in 2010.

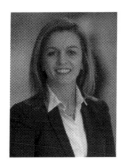

Lisiane Pruinelli, PhD, MS, RN, FAMIA is an Assistant Professor and co-director of the Center for Nursing Informatics in the School of Nursing and Affiliate Faculty at the Institute for Health Informatics, University of Minnesota. She is a Fellow of the American Medical Informatics Association and a University of Minnesota School of Nursing Global Health Scholar. She serves as the co-chair of the Nursing Knowledge Big Data Science Initiative, co-chair for the Data Science and Clinical Analytics workgroup, and as an advisor board member for the International Medical Informatics Association—Student and Emerging Professional interest group. Previously, she served as a co-chair for the Midwest Nursing Research Society Nursing Informatics workgroup. With more than ten years of clinical experience in both transplant coordination and information systems development and implementation, she is part of a new generation of nursing informaticians focused on applied clinical informatics. Her expertise is in applying innovative nursing informatics tools and cutting-edge data science methods to investigate the trajectory of complex disease conditions suitable for clinical implementations. Her work aims to identify the problems and targeted interventions for better patient outcomes. Dr. Pruinelli grew up in Brazil, moved to USA in 2012 and brings an international and diverse perspective to her everyday work and life. She earned a PhD degree from the University of Minnesota School of Nursing in 2016, and a Master's of Sciences (2008), a Teaching Degree in Nursing (2002) and a Bachelor of Nursing Sciences (2000) degree from the Federal University of Rio Grande do Sul, Porto Alegre, Brazil.

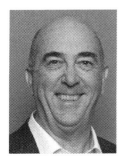

Patrick Weber, MA, RN, FIAHSI, FGBHI is Founder, Director and Principal of Nice Computing, SA in Lausanne, Switzerland. He holds a MA degree in healthcare management and is a Registered Nurse with a diploma degree in nursing. Weber has been an active leader in the European health informatics field for over 30 years, serving as his country's representative to IMIA-Nursing for over a decade and has held numerous board-level positions in IMIA-Nursing as well. Weber is an active member and leader in the European Federation for Medical Informatics (EFMI) and has held numerous leadership positions including treasurer, vice president, president and past president over the past decades. He has served as the vice president of MedInfo 2019 at International Medical Informatics Association (IMIA) and vice president

Europe, and is currently the IMIA Liaison Officer to WHO, Geneva. Within his own country, Weber leads the expert group for Swiss DRG quality control for medical coding and is President of the Oliver Moeschler Foundation leading pre-hospitalization healthcare emergencies. He is EFMI Leader of EU H2020 projects such as CrowdHealth, FAIR4Health and HosmartAI. He is the co-editor of *Nursing Informatics for the 21st Century: An International Look at Practice, Trends and Future*, first and second editions; *Nursing Informatics 2016 eHealth for All: Every Level Collaboration – From Project to Realization*; and *Forecasting Informatics Competencies for Nurses in the Future of Connected Health*. Weber is a founding member of the International Academy of Health Sciences Informatics and a member of the Board of the Swiss Medical Coding Association.

Contributors

Henry Adams, B.Comn, InterSystems Corporation, South Africa

Miriam de Abreu Almeida, PhD, RN, Full Professor, School of Nursing, Universidade Federal do Rio Grande do Sul

Robyn Begley, DNP, RN, NEA-BC, FAAN, AONL Chief Executive Officer, AHA Senior Vice President and Chief Nursing Officer, American Organization for Nursing Leadership (AONL)

Helen J. Betts, EdD, MEd (SEN), BA, PGCEA, SRN, SCM, ADM, MTD, HELINA Education Working Group

Whende M. Carroll, MSN, RN-BC, FHIMSS, Director, Clinical Optimization, Contigo Health

Catherine Chronaki, MSc, DiplEng, Secretary General, HL7 Europe Foundation

Amy Cramer, BSN, MMCi, CPHQ, Director, Global Product Development Strategic Partnerships, Pfizer Limited

Fabio D'Agostino, PhD, RN, Associate Professor of Nursing, Saint Camillus International University of Health and Medical Sciences

Rebecca Freeman, PhD, RN, FAAN, FNAP, Vice President for Health Informatics, University of Vermont Health Network

Nicholas R. Hardiker, PhD, RN, FACMI, FAAN, Professor of Nursing & Health Informatics, University of Huddersfield

Chrispin Kabuya, MSc, BSc, Walter Sisulu University

Margaret Ann Kennedy, PhD, RN, Senior Principal, Accenture, Canada

Minna Kaija-Kortelainen, MSSc, Bachelor of Law, Registered Social Worker, Senior Lecturer, Savonia University of Applied Sciences

Pirkko Kouri, PhD, PHN, RN, Finnish Society of Telemedicine and eHealth/International Society for Telemedicine & eHealth

Gerri Lamb, PhD, RN, FAAN, Edson College of Nursing and Health Innovation, Arizona State University

Julibeth Lauren, PhD, APRN, ACNS-BC, Vice-President, Practice and Clinical Education, M Health Fairview

Anne Moen, PhD, RN, FACMI, FIAHSI, Professor, Institute for Health and Society, Faculty of Medicine, University of Oslo

Aline Tsuma Gaedke Nomura, PhD, RN, Radiology Service Charge Nurse, Hospital de Clínicas de Porto Alegre

Sheila Ochylski, DNP, RN-BC, FAMIA, Chief Nurse Informatics Officer, U.S. Department of Veterans Affairs

Laura-Maria Peltonen, PhD, Docent, FEANS, Department of Nursing Science, University of Turku

Laura Reed, DNP, MBA, RN, Executive Vice President, Chief Nursing Executive, and Chief Operating Officer, M Health Fairview

Sanaz Riahi, PhD, RN, Vice President, Practice, Academics & Chief Nursing Executive, Ontario Shores Centre for Mental Health Sciences; Lecturer, Department of Psychiatry, University of Toronto

Anne W. Snowdon, PhD, RN, FAAN, Professor, Strategy and Entrepreneurship, Odette School of Business, University of Windsor

Gillian Strudwick, PhD, RN, FAMIA, Chief Clinical Informatics Officer and Scientist, Centre for Addiction and Mental Health; Assistant Professor, Institute of Health Policy, Management and Evaluation, University of Toronto

Jude L. Tayaben, PhD, RN, Assistant Professor, College of Nursing, Benguet State University

Riitta Turjamaa, PhD, PHN, RN, Manager, Savonia University of Applied Sciences and post doc researcher, Department of Nursing Science, University of Eastern Finland

Kristen K. Will, PhD, MHPE, PA-C, College of Health Solutions, Arizona State University

Graham Wright, MPhil, MBA, DN (Lon), Cert Ed, FBCS, FIAHSI, SRN, RMN, RNT, Professor Extraordinarius, University of South Africa; Chair, SAHIA Working Group, HELINA Education Working Group

Introduction

The emergence of digital health has been palpable, particularly, in the past decade. Enhanced by the pandemic, social injustices and inequities and planetary health urgency, this book explores and summarizes this evolution and the current state of digital health. Anchored in Chapter 1, Snowdon introduces digital health, beginning with the origins, evolution and definition of digital health and the pivotal role of nurses in advancing the transformation of health systems towards digital health ecosystems of tomorrow. Building on this introduction, Carroll in Chapter 2 describes 21st-century nursing care encompassing new technologies, including artificial intelligence (AI), the internet of medical things (IoMT), virtual and augmented reality and cloud computing. Carroll discusses how these technologies are transforming how nurses deliver patient, family and community care and manage operations of systems across the care continuum in the age of digital health. Strudwick, Riahi, and Hardiker bring an international lens in Chapter 3, while providing strategies and solutions to the current challenges preventing the advancement of digital health from being realized. The opportunities and challenges of digital health call for specific attention to ethics as addressed in Chapter 4. Kouri, Kaija-Kortelainen, Kennedy, and Turjamaa provide an introduction to the foundations of ethics, applications in our contemporary digital society, the ethics of technology use with older persons and a special emphasis on ownership and the patient role in creating health data.

Transformation to digital health has powerful implications for healthcare and nursing leadership in the US and globally. In Chapter 5, Begley, Reed and Lauren highlight the roles of nurse executives in the digital transformation for nursing and healthcare. The role of the nurse executive is an essential building block for patient centered care, meeting the consumer demand and the shift to non-traditional care delivery models for convenient on demand care that is connected and extends responsive services. Moen, Cramer and Chronaki add complementary specific detail in Chapter 6. Peltonen focuses in Chapter 7 on how the adoption of new technologies has the potential to improve service user, staff and organizational outcomes. Combined with the evolving roles in nursing and change in care delivery, the expectations for nursing leaders, who need to prepare themselves with a vision for the future and necessary competence for leading this change, is expansive. Appropriate strategic planning and tactical implementation of information and communication technologies to meet with future demands will aid to achieve the quadruple aim to optimize health system performance.

A broader systems perspective, including global comparisons, extends our understanding of the digital health evolution. Ochylski and Freeman in Chapter 8 provide a strong emphasis on people, process, technology and culture in this view of the history of Health IT and nursing informatics in large health systems. This chapter includes the journey of transformation of nursing informatics within the Veterans Affairs and other non-VA large healthcare systems. Together, these authors with over 50 years of healthcare experience within complex healthcare organizations and large government entities offer their vision for what nursing informatics *could be* in a large health system's drive towards organizational excellence and exemplary patient outcomes, where technology supports the best practice pathways of extraordinary care teams. D'Agostino, Almeida, Nomura, and Tayaben address global viewpoints in Chapter 9. Moreover, Wright, Bett, Kabuya and Adams summarize additional health systems transformation in Chapter 10.

Finally, digital health is pervaded with the call for teams, which Will and Lamb address in Chapter 11. Nursing and healthcare teams have demonstrated tremendous impact on clinical outcomes, provider and patient well-being while lowering healthcare costs. While nurses play a critical role in healthcare teams facilitating important teamwork processes, including communication and coordination, traditional methods of studying teams have kept integral members of the healthcare team hidden, especially for non-billable providers, such as nursing and other healthcare providers. The electronic health record, a rich source of big data which captures real-time clinical outcomes, is a tremendous resource for capturing the impact teams have on clinical outcomes and further allows for more accurate capture of team member attribution.

In summary, this book includes a current state synopsis of healthcare in the USA and global exemplars, with the inclusion of a discussion of specific implications for nursing leaders and executives. Engagement of the people (patients, families, communities) as partners in enhancing health is described. Information management and the necessary definition and access to data are discussed with a particular explication of the role of information management and operational decision making. The challenges and learnings related to informatics drawn from the experiences of leaders in large health systems shed insights into the current state of informatics enabled digital health and healthcare. The global example of the equal integration of technology, nursing and health systems expands our knowledge of the current state as well as exploring possibilities. The commitment to and description of the current state of teamwork and integral role/functions within informatics, nursing and healthcare are core. Essentially, the current state is solidly anchored in the vital role nurses have in developing, implementing, disseminating and sustaining new technologies in digital health with solid knowledge of these technologies and an innovative spirit.

Connie White Delaney
Charlotte A. Weaver
Joyce Sensmeier
Lisiane Pruinelli
Patrick Weber

Chapter 1

Digital Health Ecosystems: A Strategy for Transformation of Health Systems in the Post-Pandemic Future

Anne W. Snowdon

Contents

DOI: 10.4324/9781003054849-1

Introduction

Healthcare systems are facing unprecedented challenges, including an aging population, managing a global pandemic, persistent growth of chronic illness, workforce shortages and healthcare costs growing far beyond GDP growth in almost every country. These challenges threaten the sustainability of every global health system and may preclude the capacity of health systems to ensure equitable access and health outcomes for every global citizen. Non-communicable disease conditions continue to place growing demands on an already fragile healthcare system as 60% of Americans experience chronic health conditions and 40% have two or more conditions, costing US health systems over $3.8 trillion annually (National Centre for Chronic Disease Prevention and Health Promotion, 2021). More recently, COVID-19 and related 'long hauler' sequelae are contributing to additional chronic health conditions as people recover from the COVID-19 virus. Sustainability and equity of health systems in the post-pandemic future is a renewed priority for every country in the world.

While health systems have struggled to manage the many demands for care delivery, consumers and populations continue to place growing expectations on health systems for equitable healthcare access and outcomes, and more personalized approaches to care delivery, particularly services focused on health and wellness (Statista, 2019). Consumers are now able to connect virtually to health teams, global experts and health organizations and have access to a wide range of health services through internet-based technologies. Reliance on virtual care services offered a lifeline to many global citizens during the COVID-19 pandemic as in-person healthcare services were suspended in an effort to contain the spread of the virus. The rapid shift toward virtual care delivery has resulted in heightened expectations among consumers for access to digitally enabled care. As health systems emerge from the pandemic, there is a renewed urgency to advance digital capacity across health systems in order to support access to healthcare services, support more equitable outcomes for populations and advance health system performance and interoperability that will be required to achieve sustainability well into the future.

This heightened 'consumerization' of healthcare is emerging rapidly as individuals are empowered to make health decisions and lifestyle choices fueled and enabled by the growing market of digital tools, wearable technologies, and health 'apps' currently available in the consumer market. Yet, health systems have struggled to keep pace with the rapid evolution of digital health technologies resulting in a disconnect between the health and wellness tools consumers are using and healthcare system information infrastructure that has not achieved the technical capacity (e.g., interoperability with consumer applications) to support consumer use of these technologies. As a result, health systems have not been able to engage patients or populations meaningfully to connect them in a way that supports and enables the achievement of personal health and wellness goals. Moreover, there remains a disconnect between the disease-focused health system and what consumers now demand from health systems; a personalized system that fits with their health and wellness needs and unique life circumstances (Snowdon et al., 2014). Evidence-based care pathways today guide a variety of health services, treatments care delivery within a standardized model where there is limited, if any, ability to personalize care strategies to fit with the unique needs, values and life circumstances of every individual person, community or population. Moreover, care pathways have had a limited focus on self-management tools and technologies to meaningfully engage people in managing their health and wellness. The post-pandemic future of healthcare will need a more modernized approach, one that facilitates meaningful relationships between providers and patients in digital societies, where much of the world's population lives today, focused on approaches that support and sustain health and wellness while proactively preventing illness. A digitally enabled health system focuses on personalized care, leveraging digital technologies to deliver care that is equitable, personalized and prioritizes the overall wellness of a patient. The key to closing the gap requires offering a personalized approach to care delivery while operating within sustainable financial models that offer choice, equity and personalized health services.

This chapter provides an introduction to digital health, beginning with the origins and evolution of digital health, an analysis and definition of digital health, the four key dimensions of digital health and the role of nurses in advancing the transformation of health systems toward digital health ecosystems of tomorrow.

Evolution of Health Information Technologies

Digital health has been described as an era (Rowlands, 2019), a progression along an evolutionary pathway of information and communication technologies (ICT) in healthcare. Digital health extends well beyond adopting technologies to 'digitize' today's care delivery services. Rather, digital health constitutes a transformation of care delivery that transcends technologies to transform and modernize care delivery and health system operations. Digital health as an era is embedded in the evolutionary changes in information technology within the four industrial revolutions illustrated in Figure 1.1.

Digital health has evolved as information technologies have emerged within the four documented industrial revolutions. This represents a major shift in care delivery and mobilization of data in healthcare systems, presenting an opportunity to transform traditional provider-centric systems focused on disease management, toward a more patient-centric, proactive system focused on supporting and sustaining health and wellness. Big data, advanced analytic tools and artificial intelligence (AI) technologies are the key enablers of the 'fourth industrial evolution'—the transformation toward digital health. Although almost every other business sector has transformed its operations and delivery of services, including travel, financial services and retail, by leveraging data and analytics to improve business services, healthcare is noticeably lagging compared to other business sectors. While other sectors have embraced technology to enhance the consumer experience, healthcare has remained slow to transform established practices and

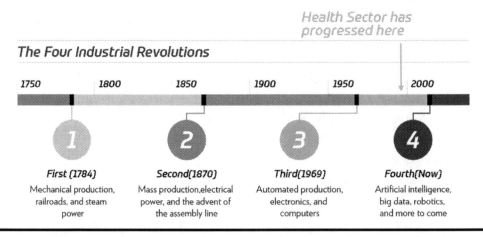

Figure 1.1   The Four Industrial Revolutions and Progress of Health Systems (adapted from Murray (2016) and Topol (2019)).

care delivery models to advance person-centric care delivery and health services that are digitally enabled.

Mainframe Computer Era (1950–1960)

Health information technology began in the early 1950s and 1960s with the introduction of mainframe computers. While mainframe computers were adopted readily by all business sectors, there was only minimal impact in the health sector. Mainframe computers advanced corporate functions in a substantive manner but had little impact on care delivery processes.

Health IT Era (1970–2000)

In the second evolutionary phase of health technology, 'Health IT' emerged as health informatics as a discipline evolved and problem-oriented health records were implemented. Over the course of this 30-year period, personal computers came into the consumer market and health IT departments advanced and deployed Enterprise IT systems to manage corporate information in health organizations, such as hospitals. The primary focus of health IT included logistics and organizational functions with a major focus on performance management systems. Examples included systems such as human resources management and finance.

By the late 1990s, the personal computer became normalized, as telecommunication networks and modern software became integrated into hospital systems (Rowlands, 2019).

eHealth Era (2000–2020)

The new millennium ushered in the era of eHealth where healthcare practices were more directly supported by communication and information technologies and computer systems and digital technology (World Health Organization, 2012). Health systems were facing substantial growth in chronic illness (e.g., non-communicable illness), which required a significant need for quality and safety data to inform care delivery.

Consumerism of healthcare has advanced dramatically since 2000 with the rapid evolution of health applications available to consumers worldwide. These were often deployed on smartphones offering consumers personalized health services 'in the palm of their hand.' This era of eHealth dramatically shifted consumer access to health information. This access continues to fuel consumer empowerment and self-management of their health and wellness. The eHealth era focused more directly on patient care delivery, whereby digital technologies were adopted to inform provider-directed care leveraging evidence-based care pathways. Likewise, e-commerce emerged during the eHealth era, focused on enterprise-wide shared health records, known as the electronic medical record (EMR), and later referred to as the Electronic Health Record. These were implemented across entire health systems. The first Electronic Healthcare Record (EHR) technologies digitized patient information, making it clearer to read and more accessible to health-care practitioners across different healthcare institutions (Evans, 2016). The eHealth era significantly advanced the emergence of consumerism in digital societies, as new telecommunications and larger bandwidths enabled health tools and applications designed directly for the consumer, that provided every person with access to personalized tools such as wearable devices and personalized health applications (Rowlands, 2019). As telecommunications boomed, so did digital phone applications (known as 'apps'), offering the opportunity for people to actively engage and manage their own health and wellness, using apps and wearable technologies available in the consumer market. The rapid advancement of digital technologies for consumers contin-ues to evolve, fueling self-management of health and wellness care, moving well beyond the traditional role of 'recipient of healthcare' typically focused on disease management, toward the role of proactive decision-maker in managing personal health goals (Rowlands, 2019).

Digital health (2020 and beyond)

Digital health is now considered an evolutionary leap that will transform healthcare systems from the provider-focused system of today, toward the digital health ecosystem of tomorrow. In this ecosystem of the future, indi-viduals and populations will be actively engaged and empowered to manage their personal health and wellness, supported by provider teams accessible within digital societies. The digital health era is enabled by the integra-tion of artificial intelligence (AI), which mobilizes big data from multiple sources (e.g., clinical data sources, personal health data sources), to support advances in predictive analytics able to proactively identify risk, and inform prevention efforts to mitigate risks and protect or sustain health and well-ness. Digital health mobilizes information technologies such as AI, robotics, machine learning, internet of things, self-help applications, virtual reality and many others. Advances in these and other technologies are anticipated to enable health system teams to participate actively in digital societies where consumer demand or need for health services can be responsive when and where care is needed, and mobilization of data from multiple sources (e.g. wearables, apps, smartphones) can be integrated into care delivery processes to support personalization of care delivery.

The era of digital health puts the person at the center, thus transforming the relationship between health and patient (Rowlands, 2019). This era makes it possible to personalize and diversify care delivery, focused on the unique needs of every individual person. In digital health, rapidly emerging information technologies will enable a strategic shift from today's reactive approach to care delivery focused on diagnosis and management of disease toward a more personalized and proactive approach to supporting health and wellness. New digital technologies and access to information delivered in the palm of the hands of the person, creating and owning their personal health data, shifts the relationship from patients who are recipients of care toward person-centric care models where health providers partner with individuals to support their health journey and life course. The digital health era places a new urgency on interoperability within and across health systems and digital societies where people participate. Interoperability will enable seamless, safe and secure integration of multiple sources of data to enable and inform personalized, data-driven decision-making across health systems.

The evolution of health and information technologies and the four eras which have now enabled the era of digital health provide an important historical context for examining digital health. Health information technologies in the digital health era now present the opportunity for an unprecedented transformation of healthcare systems. However, the many impressive opportunities for robust, high performing and personalized health systems worldwide, able to support every global citizen to realize their potential, will not be realized unless and until health system leaders, program teams, nurses and other clinician leaders, and the populations health systems serve, come together to collaborate and co-design the strategic pathways to the future, to achieve transformation of health systems into digital health ecosystems, described in the following sections.

The 'Empowered Consumer'

It has become increasingly apparent that there is a poor fit between what formal health systems have to offer (i.e., dominant disease management care pathways, 'one size fits all') and what empowered consumers value and are seeking to achieve (i.e., health and wellness). The basis for this disconnect is two-fold. First, health systems have focused primarily on managing illness and disease using prescribed care pathways, rather than focusing on individual health and wellness goals where care pathways are adapted and personalized to the unique life circumstances, values and health goals of the individual (Snowdon et al., 2014).

Second, consumers today have access to a wide variety of health services, health applications, wearables and internet-based information. Thus, consumers define and design their own strategies to support health and wellness, relying on digital tools and services in the consumer market which are independent of formalized health systems. The challenge is that the majority of digital tools and platforms available online for consumers are not connected to or interoperable with information systems in formalized health systems, making it nearly impossible for consumers to connect meaningfully to health teams and leverage digital technologies.

The growth of phone applications (apps), digital technologies and devices such as wearables (ex. Fitbit, Apple Health) has offered consumers alternative approaches to therapies and health management tools. The majority of these tools and applications enable reporting and tracking valuable information about personal health and lifestyle choices. However, these tools are not interoperable with information infrastructure in traditional health systems. One significant challenge with this lack of interoperability and connectivity is the challenge of health literacy, whereby consumers may have difficulty filtering credible health information from information which has little or no basis in objective health evidence and knowledge.

Essentially, today there are two distinct and separate healthcare systems: the traditional healthcare system, which is institution-centric (e.g., hospital dominant) and prioritizes disease management and services which are delivered in person; and the consumer-based health system, where people select and engage online health tools, wearables and resources to create their own personalized strategy to manage their health and wellness, customized to their needs, values and goals of the individual (Snowdon et al., 2014). If digital health is to advance and progress toward a system that prioritizes the health and wellness of people and populations, one must first understand the motivations of people as consumers of health services. Understanding consumer incentives toward personalized approaches to health and wellness is critical. In a 2014 study, seven key motivations or 'drivers' that fuel the empowered consumer in health systems were identified (Snowdon et al., 2014). These seven motivators are:

1. *Drive to learn and manage wellness.* People are generally averse to waiting and wondering if they will get sick before seeking healthcare services. People are motivated to learn healthy behaviors and strategies that fit with their personal health and wellness goals. People are motivated to feel good. Access to health information and the explosion in the use of health applications ('apps') is a clear indication of the thirst for health and wellness tools and technologies sought after by consumers the world over.

2. *Drive to engage and connect to others 'like me.'* People actively participate in digital societies, often engaging with other people in digital 'communities,' composed of people who share interests and values or may be experiencing similar health challenges or goals or sharing health strategies that have supported and advanced wellness. Online peer-to-peer support is offering consumer support and learning from 'people like me,' which encourages and enables progress toward shared health goals. While the validity of the medical information provided through these social networks may not be considered credible or 'evidence-based,' these are powerful networks that inform, influence and share health information and experiences.

3. *Drive for Autonomy.* People inherently strive for, and value, self-determination. What is most important and what matters in terms of their individual health and wellness journey, all fuel the drive toward autonomy, control of their own destiny and self-determination to achieve personal goals. People are no longer waiting or relying on health information from providers; they are making their own decisions, seeking information they believe offers value and accessing information online that they deem relevant to their individual needs and health circumstances.

4. *Drive to self-manage health information.* People today are seeking health information that is relevant to them, their values and their personal circumstances. Although health systems have begun to provide access to personal health data, there has been less progress toward personalized, health literacy tools that enable self-management of health, ability to report progress toward health goals and education tools that engage consumers meaningfully to manage health and wellness. While people strive toward independence and autonomy in making decisions, personalized approaches to engaging consumers and supporting self-management is less well developed in health systems.

5. *Drive for precision, accuracy and confidence in healthcare.* People who have access to, and manage their own health information are more confident in the quality of their care—as they are able to recognize and

track their progress, evaluate risks and ensure they are receiving quality care. The growing rate of medical errors has eroded confidence in health systems, with 1 in 10 people globally experiencing medical error (World Health Organization, 2019). Transparency and meaningful engagement of consumers in managing their health and wellness build confidence among consumers in the quality, safety and accuracy of care delivery.

6. *Drive to collaborate and partner with health providers.* Empowering with access to information from both the consumer and the provider creates an opportunity for meaningful connectivity and engagement between the person and their health provider team(s), creating the conditions for shared decision-making. Digital technologies offer the potential to transform the traditional 'in-person' visits with providers toward a more digitally enabled care environment that offers convenience, choice and opportunity for personalization.

7. *Drive toward consumer engagement.* The phenomenon of 'Dr Google' is more than just the availability of, and access to, online technology. Responding to the trend of the empowered consumer is challenging for health systems as it undermines the hegemony of the medical model of health, where there are established traditions of professional judgments of clinical 'need' be considered above the 'wants,' 'preferences' or 'choices' of patients. Healthcare consumerism is about enabling people to self-manage their health, fueled by the fundamental value of self-determination of what it means to be human.

Defining Digital Health

A variety of terms and concepts are used interchangeably when describing or referencing digital health, including 'mHealth' (mobile health), 'eHealth' (e.g., technology and digital applications to assist patients in their health), virtual care and telehealth, to name just a few. A concept analysis of digital health definitions in both empirical literature and grey literature (e.g., online sources) reveals three dominant themes that underpin how digital health is defined.

Digital Health is Defined in Terms of the Type and Use of Digital Technologies

The most prevalent focus of digital health definitions in current publications focuses on the type and use of digital technologies in healthcare

(Gardiner, 2019; Canada Health Infoway, 2020; Lupton, 2014; Robinson et al., 2015; Scotland Digital Health Institute, 2018; WHO, 2019). For example, 'Digital Health is a term that is frequently adopted to encompass a wide range of technologies related to health and medicine' (Lupton, 2014).

Similarly, 'digital health refers to the use of information technology/ electronic communication tools, services, and processes to deliver healthcare services' (Canada Health Infoway, 2020). These definitions, most common in the literature, limit the defining features of digital health in terms of the use of specific technologies and limit digital health as a concept to a focus on technologies, rather than a focus or definition of digital health in terms of what it can achieve and for who.

Digital Health Definitions Focused on Improvement of Healthcare Delivery

A number of definitions focus on the use of digital technologies to improve the delivery of healthcare, such as improving the holistic view of patients (FDA); 'achieving health objectives' (UNICEF, 2018); upgrading the practice of medicine (Steinhubl & Topol, 2018); delivering evidence-based therapeutic interventions to prevent, manage, or treat a disease or disorder (Goldsack et al., 2019); monitor and improve wellbeing and health of patients (Iyawa et al., 2016); measure and intervene to support human health (Best, 2019); improve health system performance and capacity to deliver care, treat patients, track diseases and monitor public health (Deloitte, 2019; European Society of Cardiology, 2019; Swiss Tropical and Public Health Institute, 2020). These definitions define the use of digital technologies as a strategy to optimize or advance existing care delivery strategies to strengthen the management and treatment of diseases and outcomes of care delivery.

Digital Health as a Strategy for Health System Transformation

Less common but very compelling are more recent definitions of digital health focusing on system transformation toward patient-centric, democratization of care. Specifically, Trono (2016) defines digital health as a revolution that enables medicine to transform from a 'reactive and often empirical discipline' into a 'precise, preventive, personalized and participatory endeavor.' Mesko et al. (2017) describe the 'cultural transformation of how disruptive technologies provide digital and objective data accessible to both caregivers and patients, leading to an equality in doctor-patient relationship with shared decision-making and democratization of care.' Rowlands (2019) defines digital health within the context of digital societies whereby

> data is harvested in real-time across all societal activities, sophisticated analyses distill knowledge from these data to encourage better health and better value by including a wide range of economic activities and technologies. In this definition, healthcare is citizen-centric, decentralized and requires health providers to participate, not control.

This key theme of citizen-centric and the empowerment of individuals has gained attention by a number of regulatory organizations (FDA, 2018), researchers (Iyawa et al., 2016) and professional societies (Goldsack et al., 2019).

The digital health era reflects transformation of healthcare toward an ecosystem, a new architecture and collaborative environment that extends well beyond digitizing today's health system. Digital health proposes an interactive and dynamic community full of rich data and information sharing that is cross-disciplinary in learning and flexibility (Chang & West, 2006; Heintzman, 2015). The definition of digital health first published by HIMSS (Healthcare Information and Management Systems Society, Inc) advances and informs the transformation of health systems worldwide to advance and support the full realization of health by every human everywhere, defined as follows:

> Digital health connects and empowers people and populations to manage health and wellness, augmented by accessible and supportive provider teams working within flexible, integrated, interoperable and digitally enabled care environments that strategically leverage digital tools, technologies and services to transform care delivery.

(Snowdon, 2019)

The evolution of digital health as a concept is evident in the thematic review of definitions which offer a glimpse into digital health as an opportunity to transform healthcare systems from a provider-centric model where patients are recipients of care, to digital health ecosystems that empower people to manage their health and wellness, leveraging the digital infrastructure and technology to support and inform health decisions, focused on supporting and sustaining health and wellness, whereby care teams are partners in care engaged in shared decision-making.

Digital health, also referred to as an ecosystem, a new architecture and collaborative care environment that extends beyond traditional human reach; provides an interactive community, rich data and information, value-add customer and agent services, high connectivity, cross-disciplinary learning and flexibility; and orients around self-empowerment of users (Chang & West, 2006; Janjua et al., 2009; Heintzman, 2015).

Digital Health Frameworks and Concepts

Current digital health frameworks and models offer insights into the concepts that are associated with digital health across the published digital health frameworks. Key themes of digital health concepts were analyzed across all published digital health models and frameworks described in the literature. The concepts central to digital health become clear—including governance and leadership, data infrastructure, analytics, person-enabled healthcare and a focus on outcomes at the system level. Based on an analysis of current digital health frameworks, four key dimensions of digital health emerge, defined in the following section (Snowdon, 2019).

Person-enabled healthcare is the prioritization of healthcare services that support people and populations to manage their health and wellness within the context of their personal values, needs and unique life circumstances. Person-enabled health is a hallmark feature of digital health described across a number of models and frameworks, which places the individual at the center of health and wellness care.

Predictive analytics is the transformation of data into information, knowledge and insights, to create real-world evidence to inform decisions. Health systems generate massive amounts of data. However, unless data is mobilized, exchanged and analyzed to reveal insights, information and knowledge, it cannot adequately inform stakeholder decisions (e.g., individual decisions and provider decisions) to achieve health and wellness. Predictive analytics contribute to 'learning' health systems, whereby robust analytics track health outcomes for unique population segments to enable systems to learn and define the care delivery strategies that achieve best outcomes and the conditions under which best outcomes are achieved for every individual and population.

Governance and workforce is the system-level strategy that guides the implementation of digital health across global health systems. Governance ensures the policy and regulatory environment of health systems guards privacy, security, stewardship and accountability. Strongly linked to performance and strategy is the integrity, capacity and sustainability of the health workforce, which is critical to ensuring people and populations have secure connectivity to care teams, and data is accessible across the journey of care.

Digital Health Ecosystems

The definition of digital health and the four dimensions of digital health have emerged from a concept analysis of published definitions, models and frameworks of digital health (Snowdon, 2019). It is particularly clear in the literature that authors distinguish the role of 'patients' as recipients of care, in today's healthcare systems, from the role of the person, a role defined by choice, expectation and empowerment (Rowlands, 2019) that reflects and aligns with digital health ecosystems. The role of the consumer is one of many roles that an individual may assume in digital health systems. Digital health shifts the priorities of healthcare delivery from a dominant focus on disease management toward a focus on health and wellness across the life journey. Disease management remains a necessary and important role in digital health. However, engaging and enabling a person to self-manage their health, and disease condition(s) in a preventive and proactive approach is the priority focus of a digital health ecosystem. Each of the following four dimensions of digital health ecosystems is described in the following section.

Person-enabled Healthcare

Person-enabled health is defined as a health system focused on meeting and delivering on individual needs, values and personalized health goals. In digital health, we suggest the use of the term 'person' over patient, as the term 'patient' suggests that individuals are viewed as 'recipients' of care. In digital health ecosystems, the individual is seen as a person, the primary decision-maker and manager of their own health and wellness. Person-enabled healthcare recognizes the value and importance of meaningful relationships between people and their care teams, creating a partnership based on individual needs, choice and trust. Digital tools and technologies enable people to track their progress toward their personal health and wellness goals, while engaging with health teams as partners, supporting and informing their decisions and offering options and choices, to strengthen health literacy and enable evidence-informed health decisions. When people are engaged and empowered to manage their own health and wellness, care pathways are leveraged to inform care options that are then personalized to individual needs and circumstances to achieve improved healthcare outcomes (Milani et al., 2017; Hibbard et al., 2004). Each person engages in self-management of their health to varying degrees, based on their unique life circumstances, values, as well as the complexity of health conditions and health status (Milani et al., 2017). Effective digital health approaches to care delivery profiles how health services can be personalized to each individual, based on engagement and complexity of health status. There are three features of person-enabled care described in the following:

1. *Personalized care delivery:* The personalization of care, where the person is the decision-maker, managing their care, tracking progress toward personal health goals leveraging digital tools and technologies (e.g., personal digital tools, mobile devices, wearables) the person chooses that best suit their unique life circumstances and personalized approaches to healthcare. Care providers partner with the person to support and inform decisions, characterized by shared decision-making, focused on advancing progress toward personal health goals.
2. *Proactive risk management:* Focuses on care delivery that proactively identifies risks to health and wellness, cues individuals and their provider teams of the risks and strategies to inform proactive interventions to prevent risk and sustain or strengthen progress toward health goals. This dimension of digital health prioritizes proactive risk management to prevent illness or disease exacerbations, personalized to the unique health goals of each individual. It is a shift from the siloed, reactive disease management approach of today's health systems, to one of proactive, seamless integration of services that prevent illness, support health, wellness and quality of life.
3. *Predictive population health*: Health system data is mobilized to track population health outcomes to evaluate progress toward health, wellness and quality of life across the life course. Population health identifies and anticipates risks and equity of health outcomes to inform program strategies or models of care focused on managing and reducing risks to health for each unique population segment a health system is mandated to serve. Examples of this population health approach

include proactively tracking health and wellness progress and outcomes for unique segments such as rural communities, indigenous peoples, vulnerable populations (e.g., homeless, financial insecurity, food insecurity), children, seniors, essential workers and so on. Predictive population health is informed by a robust analytics infrastructure that mobilizes digital tools, dashboards and public reporting strategies to inform health services and programs aimed at strengthening population health outcomes.

Each of these dimensions focuses on the personalization of care for every person, meaningful and supportive relationships between every person and their health provider teams, and proactive care delivery to optimize health and wellness of unique populations, leveraging digital tools and technologies to track progress toward health outcomes, track equity (e.g., of outcomes and access to care) to inform personalized care delivery focused on health and wellness.

Predictive Analytics

Data and analytics are foundational tools in digital health ecosystems. The use of data and information makes real-time decision-making possible, using analytics to distill information, knowledge and insights from the data, creating predictive strategies that generate better health and value (Rowlands, 2019). Health systems are generating massive amounts of data (Rowlands, 2019), but the data must be mobilized safely and securely, analyzed without bias and translated into knowledge and information. Predictive analytics is defined as the transformation of data into knowledge and real-world insights that inform decisions for individuals, communities and populations in partnership with health teams, and health system leaders. As rapidly expanding sources and volumes of data become available, it brings with it new opportunities to generate knowledge, insights and information (Carvalho et al., 2019).

Predictive analytics makes it possible for systems to learn what care works best, for who and under what conditions best outcomes are achieved. Predictive analytics brings together health system data, along with personal digital tools and applications, population data, to inform care delivery and operations, that inform care delivery that is proactive, informed by prediction of risk to optimize health outcomes, to support health and well-ness. Predictive analytics has three sub-dimensions:

1. *Personalized analytics*: Personalized analytics collects individual health and wellness data from multiple sources (e.g., personal digital tools, applications, mobile devices, wearables), including 'progressive' data sources (e.g., social, genomic and biometric), to enable individuals and their provider teams to track progress toward health and wellness goals at the individual level.

2. *Predictive Analytics:* Predictive analytics track and trace outcomes across the journey of care for every individual patient, to identify outcomes that work best for every individual and the conditions under which best outcomes are achieved. Predictive analytics also tracks program and population-level outcomes, equity of outcomes across population segments and programs to identify risk for potential harm or poor outcomes. Predictive analytics offers a proactive view of health system outcomes within and across population segments which generates the evidence to inform care delivery strategies that strengthen quality and safety outcomes.

3. *Operational analytics.* Operational analytics mobilizes data from multiple sources (health services, patient-reported outcomes, adverse events, workforce) to track health system performance outcomes including, but not limited to, efficiency, productivity, workflow, safety, quality, workforce capacity and sustainability, supply and logistics outcomes and financial performance. Operational analytics use digital tools and dashboards to track operational outcomes to evaluate progress toward strategic goals, such as financial sustainability, equity, quality and effectiveness of care program outcomes and personalization of care delivery in advancing population health and wellness. The use of digital tools and dashboards inform leadership, operations and governance bodies' decisions.

Each of these dimensions contributes to analytics capacity that creates the evidence of value and outcomes relevant to health system performance to identify care processes and health services that offer best outcomes for every individual and population segment, offering continuous feedback in real-time to monitor and create transparency of outcomes, to inform decisions across the health system and populations they are mandated to serve.

Governance and Workforce

Governance and workforce are essential to digital health ecosystems, providing the leadership and accountability required to support a robust and high-performing digital health ecosystem. Governance and workforce are defined as the strategic leadership and oversight of digital health systems that support the policy and regulatory environment of health systems, including privacy, security, stewardship and accountability. Principles of strong digital health governance are important for data stewardship, data integrity, workforce sustainability, equity, diversity and inclusion. This includes principles of confidentiality and accountability, transparency, policy and decision-making processes that are well-informed and accountable, advance equity and inclusiveness and enables individual engagement (Marcelo et al., 2017; Benedict & Schlieter, 2015)

Governance prioritizes a focus on a sustainable, high-performing workforce that is prepared and supported to deliver digitally enabled health services working within highly automated and optimized work environments. The future of sustainable, high-performing digital health ecosystems requires unique governance structures to transform workplace environments that make it possible for providers to support people to manage their health and wellness, engage meaningfully with providers as partners, re-designing care models to prioritize health and wellness across the life course for individuals and populations. Currently, leadership assumes a critical role in overcoming the current barriers to digital health. These barriers include the inconsistent use of data standards, inconsistent application of policies, siloed health information systems, care delivery models reliant on in-person care where patients are the recipients of care, digital platforms and technologies that are not interoperable and IT systems that do not interface or work together. Digital health requires visionary leadership that creates the conditions for the health workforce to thrive and enable optimized care environments that are automated and focused on the delivery of care rather than the management of digital technology. Accountability frameworks incentivize best care outcomes, enabled by robust digital environments that support nurses, physicians, therapists and other providers to prioritize meaningful relationships with individuals, communities and populations focused on managing health, wellness and quality of life. There are four sub-dimensions for Governance and workforce:

1) *Data stewardship.* Stewardship describes the leadership, culture, vision and objectives required to support digital health (Rosenbaum, 2010). It includes the accountability frameworks and management processes

focused on advancing the key dimensions of digital health ecosystems, aligned to the resources and workforce expertise to re-design and transform care toward personalized, proactive care approaches focused on health and wellness. Data stewardship ensures the privacy, security of data capture and mobilization and the use of analytics tools and technologies that mitigate the risk of bias to advance and strengthen the equity of outcomes and access for populations served by every health system.

2) *Policy and Decision-Making Processes.* Policy and decision-making processes include the culture and workplace environments informed by measurement of outcomes, and learning what care delivery models and approaches achieve best outcomes and the conditions under which best outcomes are achieved. Data and evidence-rich environments inform decisions on resource allocation, and governance processes guided by policy and evidence to inform strategy, and priorities to advance digital health transformation. Policy and decision-making processes include evidence-informed digital health strategy, alignment of digital care environments with personalization and person-enabled care delivery focused on achieving value, supported by health system incentives and decision-making frameworks focused on outcomes.

3) *Transparency:* Digital health systems rely on meaningful relationships between clinicians and individuals managing their health conditions, informed by data and outcomes leveraging digital tools to track progress toward health goals. Meaningful relationships are supported by consistent, transparent and verifiable communication with every individual, community and population. Health ecosystems rely on transparency to build and sustain trust and confidence of the people and communities, engaging actively in the digital societies people participate in, and/or engaging and communicating in person based on personal choice and values. Communication in digital health ecosystems focuses and prioritizes transparency of quality, safety and performance outcomes, aimed at building and sustaining user confidence in the performance of the health system. Every person is considered a partner in healthcare whereby governance and oversight ensure transparency of data sharing, people own their personal health data and may choose to share personal health information with provider teams. Dynamic engagement between providers and people managing their health supports establishing personal health goals, tracking and reporting progress toward health and wellness outcomes. Data accuracy is verified, is

accessible, equitable and transparent, while also secure and private, to ensure every individual has confidence in data and information that is communicated clearly and openly to achieve transparency.

4) *Workforce Capacity and Competency*: The rapid evolution of digital health ecosystems requires a workforce that is knowledgeable, highly skilled with access to resources to transform care delivery models and care processes from the disease management pathways of today, toward digitally enabled systems focused on supporting people and populations to manage and strengthen their health. Digitally enabled health systems require transforming digital work environments to support health providers to engage meaningfully with people, informed by automated and seamless access to data, digital tools and analytics that mobilize data and evidence to inform decisions. The future health workforce must have the resources and expertise to support and enable adoption of digital health strategies and digitally enabled models of care that support person-enabled care focused on health and wellness (Topol, 2019). Workforce policies have the accountability frameworks that support and retain a high-performing workforce that is incentivized to design, adopt and scale digitally enabled care processes and operational strategies focused on outcomes, value and impact for people, populations and operational performance that advances health system sustainability.

Governance and workforce are an essential dimension of digital health ecosystems. Without the visionary leadership to set the strategic priorities and policy frameworks to enable and support a high-performing workforce, the transformational shift toward person-enabled health and wellness will be slow and challenging to advance and achieve.

Interoperability

The fourth and final dimension of digital health ecosystems is interoperability, which has long been considered a critical infrastructure capacity of health systems to enable data to be seamlessly mobilized from multiple sources, including both formalized health data sources and user-generated sources of health data. Interoperability is the ability of different information systems, devices and applications to access, exchange, integrate and cooperatively use data in a coordinated manner, providing timely and seamless access and portability to data and information to optimize the health and wellness of individuals and populations. Connectivity means connecting all stakeholders within health organizations (between programs and departments) and across separate, autonomous, organizations within or across health systems (from one healthcare system to another) (Global Digital Health Partnership, 2019).

Interoperability focuses on the use of digital technologies to transform health systems to enable future digital health ecosystems that connect and empower people to manage their personal health and wellness journey across the life course. There are many challenges to healthcare interoperability, as many nations use different health data standards and different countries and territories are in different states of adaptation and maturity (Global Digital Health Partnership, 2019). Further, many healthcare systems vary widely in their progress toward digital maturity levels, and individuals engage and interact with many health organizations, online health services and applications, which requires the digital architecture to be able to capture, mobilize and share health data accurately and securely. The seamless flow of data requires connected, integrated, safe and secure data exchange and sharing and oversight to ensure data can be mobilized and shared with every individual. The exchange and mobilization of data across various EHR platforms and information architectures is one of the current challenges for many health systems. Addressing this challenge is critical to enable every individual to share their personal health data with providers, accurately and securely to achieve interoperability (Global Digital Health Partnership, 2019). Interoperability in a digital health ecosystem requires data standards to enable the portability of data and automated exchange of information and data to protect data ownership for every individual, and to protect their ability to choose to share data with provider teams when and where needed to support their health and wellness journey. There are four subdimensions of interoperability:

1) *Foundational Interoperability* establishes the inter-connectivity requirements needed for one system or application to securely communicate data to, and receive data from, another. Foundational interoperability ensures seamless flow of data between health organizations, systems and personal health technologies or tools.
2) *Structural Interoperability* describes the flow of data and information that is automated and integrated across multiple and varied sources of data, data reporting tools and access functions, data center structure, data integrity and information exchange. The reduction of silos of data

and information is needed to create 'visibility' of data across health systems (Global Digital Health Partnership, 2019). Structural interoperability is a key sub-dimension that supports data access and integration to overcome data silos to achieve equity in access to data.

3) *Semantic Interoperability* provides the common underlying models and codification of the data providing shared understanding and meaning to the user. Semantic interoperability leverages data standards that are open-sourced and vendor-agnostic to ensure data can be understood and communicated accurately to any global health system, in a standardized format. Interoperability based on open-sourced standards facilitates the portability of data that can be shared with providers or health organizations worldwide.

4) *Organizational Interoperability* includes governance, policy, social, legal and organizational features of data architecture that facilitate the secure, seamless and timely communication, use and sharing of data between provider teams and individuals managing their health and wellness. Organizational interoperability includes policy frameworks that ensure privacy and security of data, supports individuals to own their personal health data, and share their data when and how the individual decides to do so. Organization policy also includes accountability frameworks that guide data integrity, use of data, processes for data sharing and managing the legacy technologies to support and incentivize interoperability worldwide.

Interoperability is a key dimension of digital health ecosystems, which makes it possible for individuals and populations to own and manage their personal health data, support credentialing of data to make it portable and able to be shared with providers when needed. Interoperability standards ensure a common 'language' of data that is standardized to ensure every individual, every provider team and every health system globally is able to access data to inform care decisions.

The Role of Nurses in Digital Health Ecosystems

The evolution of digital health ecosystems is advancing and may well have been accelerated by the global COVID-19 pandemic. Never before has there been a greater urgency for digital health ecosystems that engage populations and individuals meaningfully, to support self-management of health and wellness, connected and supported by provider teams as partners in care. Throughout the pandemic, global citizens were challenged to manage their health and disease conditions, and self-manage the risks of COVID-19, without meaningful or well-established digital tools and connectivity to health systems. Citizens worldwide were challenged to find credible, objective data and evidence to inform their day-to-day decisions to guard against infection with the COVID-19 virus and manage their unique health needs and life circumstances.

There is now an urgency as health systems are challenged to manage to test for surveillance of the pandemic, track vaccinations and rates of infection with limited interoperability and few health systems able to digitally optimize care delivery from public health to primary care, acute care and community-based care in the home. The early waves of the pandemic severely restricted access to care due to the suspension of health services to mitigate the transmission of the virus in care settings. Virtual care was mobilized rapidly, which essentially digitized in-person visits with providers. However, virtual visits often precluded that the ability to share and exchange health data with interoperability between patients and their provider teams to inform decisions.

The future, post-pandemic health system must transform and re-design models of care delivery to move beyond digitizing today's healthcare delivery models, toward transforming care approaches to enable and empower people and populations to manage their health and wellness with digitally enabled tools and technologies connected to provider teams. Digital health ecosystems are revolutionizing healthcare delivery, enabling providers, particularly nurses to re-design care delivery that meaningfully connects people to their provider teams, enables integration of personal health data and clinical data generated in formal health settings to personalize care focused on the unique circumstances of every individual and population.

Nurses are uniquely positioned to lead digital health ecosystem transformation given their unique role in health systems and the unique domains of knowledge informed by theoretical frameworks and concepts that guide nursing practice focusing on whole-person care. Nursing education and research have, for decades, documented and created the evidence base for person-centric care, which is central to digital health, the hallmark of digital health ecosystems. Nursing care acknowledges what it means to be a person, and well-established nursing practices are based on empathy, caring and understanding patient experience (Weston, 2020). Nurses continuously analyze, synthesize and evaluate gathered information using experience, reflection, reasoning and observation (Weston, 2020). The experiences and expertise of nurses offer a foundation of the essential knowledge base required to transform care delivery from the disease management pathways of today, toward the personalized models of care that enable people and populations to manage their health and wellness in the post-pandemic future.

Building on the knowledge of whole-person care, nurses are the largest and the only workforce delivering care 24/7, unlike any other health professional. Nursing practice and patient care routines focused on the person, not just the disease, are foundational to re-thinking and re-designing new models of care that prioritize health literacy, the engagement and empowerment of people and their support network to manage their health and wellness, selecting digital tools and technologies that best suit their needs, values and unique life circumstances. Nurses practice from the person at the center of care, can transform care routines and practices that are commonly delivered in person, toward digitally enabled care models and approaches focused on supporting and strengthening the person's knowledge and skills to set personal goals, manage their health data and track and report progress toward personal health goals.

Technology allows and enables standards of care and ethically guiding principles used in traditional healthcare, but it is now coupled with digital technology that is transforming how care is delivered (Barbosa, 2021). Nurses' experience and expertise in care delivery are now well positioned to design digitally enabled models of care delivery that create a digital environment where meaningful relationships with individuals and their caregiver networks are able to thrive and offer care when and where needed to advance health and wellness outcomes. Artificial Intelligence (AI) offers the opportunity to aggregate very large data sets, and transform data into knowledge and richness of information (Weston, 2020) to inform proactive and preventive care approaches focused and prioritized on keeping people well. Advanced analytics can be coupled with best-practice solutions and patient-unique data, further empowering nurses to design customized care for every individual patient and family (Weston, 2020). Digital transformation offers tools and technologies to support clinical decision-making focused on supporting and sustaining health while offering ways to measure quality, safety and best practice in clinical decisions. Weston (2020) describes digital health as a way to transform nursing from transactional care delivery toward solution-based care, where data and information are mobilized by digital health ecosystems to inform proactive decisions, guided by experience and expertise in person-centric care, fueled by the automation and optimization of digital care environments.

The maturity of digital health systems creates an opportunity to transform healthcare. However, nurses must develop specific skills (Lapao, 2020) in leading transformation, co-designing digitally enabled care models with patients and their families, while at the same time working collaboratively with digital health experts in information systems, data architecture and interoperability to ensure digital work environments support excellence in care delivery. As digital health ecosystems continue to evolve, nurses are well positioned to leverage new technologies, transform digitally enabled care delivery to enable every global citizen to safely and confidently manage their health and wellness in partnership with their care providers.

To date, digital technologies and advances have focused primarily on digitizing information and data capture, and more recently digitizing in-person care visits using virtual care. To advance digital health ecosystems, nurses must have the resources and educational support to learn and develop new knowledge and skills in digital health to ensure advances in digital health ecosystems remain steadfastly focused on creating meaningful relationships between every global citizen and the providers to support their health and wellness. Nurses are often the primary professionals acting as a bridge between the health system and the patient, advocating and supporting person-centric care, translating data and knowledge into health literacy tools to support patient-centric care (McBride, 2005). The rising prevalence of chronic disease and shortages of healthcare workers, geographic spread, and health disparities create challenges in healthcare that digital health can advance and overcome (Jedamzik, 2019) as digital health ecosystem transformation advances in the post-pandemic future of healthcare.

Summary

Digital health is the evolution phase of healthcare, transforming the traditional healthcare system that is focused primarily on disease management, to one that is proactive, focused on keeping people healthy and well. This shift will require the bridging of two health systems, the traditional in which the power is currently held in the hands of administration and clinicians, and the consumer-based system, where the individual owns all of their health data, mobilizing data from both personal and form health system sources. The four dimensions of digital health transformation and interdependent, person-centered, analytics, interoperability, governance and workforce, collectively offer a roadmap to digital health transformation. They provide a framework for healthcare systems and organizations to begin their transformation to a new digital future. Through embracing the digital health revolution, healthcare systems can transform, creating sustainable healthcare systems while improving the quality and care for every global citizen everywhere to realize their full health potential.

References

Barbosa, S. de F. F. (2021). Nursing in the digital health era. *Journal of Nursing Scholarship*, 53(1), pp.5–6. https://doi.org/info:doi/

Benedict, M. & Schlieter, H. (2015). *Governance guidelines for digital healthcare ecosystems* [online]. Available at: https://www.ncbi.nlm.nih.gov/pubmed/26063282 (Accessed 22 August 2021).

Best, J. (2019, February). *What is digital health? Everything you need to know about the future of healthcare*. Retrieved from: https://www.zdnet.com/article/what-is-digital-health/

Canada Health Infoway. (2020, January). *What is digital health?* [online]. Available at: https://www.infoway-inforoute.ca/en/what-we-do/benefits-of-digital-health/what-isdigital-health (Accessed 22 August 2021).

Carvalho, J., Rocha, A., Vasconcelos, J. & Abreu, A. (2019). A health data analytics maturity model for hospitals information systems. *International Journal of Information Management*, 46, pp.278–285.

Chang, E. & West, M. (2006). *Digital ecosystems a next generation of the collaborative environment* [online]. Available at: https://pdfs.semanticscholar.org/3d08/bad6a7d379a049639eb28440a42fdd5af704.pdf (Accessed 22 August 2021).

Deloitte. (2019). *The future is here*. Retrieved from: https://www2.deloitte.com/us/en/pages/life-sciences-and-health-care/articles/healthcare-workforce-technology.html

Digital Health and Care Institute. (2018). *Digital health and care* [online]. Available at: https://www.dhi-scotland.com/about-dhi/what-is-digital-health-and-care/ (Accessed 22 August 2021).

European Society of Cardiology. (2019). *About digital health*. Retrieved from: https://www.escardio.org/Education/Digital-Health-and-Cardiology/about-digital-health

Evans, R. S. (2016 May 20). Electronic health records: Then, now, and in the future. *Yearbook of Medical Informatics*, 25(Suppl 1), pp.S48–S61. https://doi.org/10.15265/IYS-2016-s006

Food and Drug Administration. (2018). *Digital health innovation action plan* [online]. Available at: https://www.fda.gov/media/106331/download (Accessed 25 August 2021).

Gardiner, R. (2019). *Defining digital health* [online]. Available at: https://www.lsx-leaders.com/blog/what-is-digital-health (Accessed 26 August 2021).

Global Digital Health Partnership. (2019). *Connected health: Empowering health through interoperability* [online]. Available at: https://s3-ap-southeast-2.amazonaws.com/ehq-productionaustralia/57f9a51462d5e3f07569 d55232fc-c11290b99cd6/ (Accessed 29 August 2021).

Goldsack, J., Coder, M., Fitzgerald, C., Navar-Mattingly, N., Corvos, A. & Atreja, A. (2019, November). *Digital health, digital medicine, digital therapeutics (DTx): What's the difference?* Retrieved from: https://www.healthxl.com/blog/digital-health-digital-medicine-digital-therapeutics-dtx-whats-the-difference

Heintzman, N. (2015). A digital ecosystem of diabetes data and technology: Services, systems, and tools enabled by wearables, sensors, and apps. *Journal of Science and Technology*, 10(1), pp.35–41.

Hibbard, J. H., Stockard, J., Mahoney, E. R. & Tusler, M. (2004). Development of the patient activation measure (PAM): Conceptualizing and measuring activation in patients and consumers. *Health Services Research*, 39(4), pp.1005–1026.

Iyawa, G., Herselman, M. & Botha, A. (2016). Digital health innovation ecosystems: From systematic literature review to conceptual framework. *Procedia Computer Science*, 100, pp.244–252.

Janjua, N., Huddain, M., Afzal, M. & Ahmad, H. (2009). Digital health care ecosystem: SOA compliant HL7 based health care information interchange. In: 2009 3rd IEEE International Conference on Digital Ecosystems and Technologies. Retrieved from: https://ieeexplore.ieee.org/stamp/stamp.jsp?tp=&arnumber=5276681

Jedamzik, S. (2019). Digitale Gesundheit und Pflege. *Unfallchirurg*, 122, pp.670–675. https://doi.org/10.1007/s00113-019-0672-2

Lapao (2020). The nursing of the future: Combining digital health and the leadership of nurses. *Editorial Rev. Latino-Am. Enfermagem*, 28(2020). https://doi.org/10.1590/1518-8345.0000.3338

Lupton, D. (2014). Critical perspectives on digital health technologies. *Sociology Compass*, 8(12), pp.1344–1359.

Marcelo, A., Medeiros, D., Ramesh, K., Roth, S. & Wyatt, P. (2017). Transforming health systems through good digital health governance. *Asian Development Bank* [online]. Available at: https://www.adb.org/sites/default/files/publication/401976/sdwp-051-transforming-health-systems.pdf (Accessed 22 August 2021).

McBride, A. B. (2005). Nursing and the informatics revolution. *Nursing Outlook*, 53(4), pp.183–191.

Mesko, B., Drobni, Z., Benyei, E., Gergely, B. & Gyorffy, Z. (2017). Digital health is a cultural transformation of traditional healthcare. *mHealth*, 3(38). https://doi.org/10.21037/mhealth.2017.08.07

Milani, R., Lavie, C., Bober, R., Milani, A. & Ventura, H. (2017). Improving hypertension control and patient engagement using digital tools. *The American Journal of Medicine*, 130(1), pp.14–20.

Murray, A. (2016). *CEOs: The revolution is coming.* Retrieved from: https://fortune.com/2016/03/08/davos-new-industrial-revolution/

National Centre for Chronic Disease Prevention and Health Promotion. (2021). *Chronic diseases in America. Centres for disease control and prevention (CDC)* [online]. Available from: https://www.cdc.gov/chronicdisease/resources/info-graphic/chronic-diseases.htm (Accessed 28 August 2021).

Robinson, L., Griffiths, M., Wray, J., Ure, C. M. & Stein-Hodgins, J. (2015). The use of digital health technology and social media to support breast cancer. In: *Digital Mammography: A Holistic Approach.* Springer, pp.105–111.

Rosenbaum, S. (2010). Data governance and stewardship: Designing data steward-ship entities and advancing data access. *Health Services Research*, 45(5 Pt 2), pp.1442–1455. https://doi.org/10.1111/j.1475-6773.2010.01140.x

Rowlands, D. (2019, December). *What is digital health and why does it matter?* [online]. Available at: https://www.hisa.org.au/wp-content/uploads/2019/12/What_is_Digital_Health. pdf?x97063 (Accessed 22 August 2021).

Snowdon, A. (2019). *Digital health: A framework for health transformation* [online]. Available at: https://cloud.emailhimss.org/digital-health-a-framework-for-healthcare-transformation?_ga=2.143089971.76683002.1629031413-1151317647.1629031412 (Accessed 22 August 2021).

Snowdon, A., Schnarr, K. & Alessi, C (2014). *"It's All About Me": The personalization of health systems* [online]. Available at: https://www.ivey.uwo.ca/cmsmedia/3467873/its-all-about-me-the-personalizationof-health-systems.pdf (Accessed 22 August 2021).

Statista. (2019, October). *Global digital population as of October 2019.* Retrieved from: Statista: https://www.statista.com/statistics/617136/digital-population-worldwide/

Steinhubl, S. & Topol, E. (2018). Digital medicine, on its way to being just plain medicine. *NPJ Digital Medicine*, (1), p.20175.

Swiss Tropical and Public Health Institute. (2020). *Digital health.* Retrieved from: https://www.swisstph.ch/en/topics/health-systems-and-interventions/digital-health/

Topol, E. (2019). *The Topol report: Preparing the healthcare workforce to deliver the digital future* [online]. Available at: https://www.hee.nhs.uk/our-work/topol-review (Accessed 22 August 2021).

Trono, D. (2016). Switzerland and the digital health revolution. *Life Sciences in Switzerland*, 70(12), pp.851–852.

UNICEF. (2018). *UNICEF's approach to digital health* [online]. Available at: https://www.unicef.org/innovation/media/506/file/UNICEF%27s%20Approach%20to%20Digital%20Health%E2%80%8B%E2%80%8B.pdf (Accessed 22 August 2021).

Weston, M. (2020). Nursing practice in the digital age. *Nurse Leader*, 18(3), pp.286–289. https://doi.org/10.1016/j.mnl.2020.03.004

World Health Organization. (2012). *National eHealth strategy toolkit* [online]. Available at: https://www.who.int/ehealth/publications/overview.pdf (Accessed 22 August 2021).

World Health Organization. (2019). *Who guideline recommendations on digital interventions for health system strengthening: Executive summary* [online]. Available at: https://apps.who.int/iris/bitstream/ handle/10665/311977/WHO-RHR-19.8-eng.pdf?ua=1 (Accessed 22 August 2021).

Chapter 2

Digital Health and New Technologies

Whende M. Carroll

Contents

DOI: 10.4324/9781003054849-2

Overview of New Technologies in Healthcare and Nursing

Definition of New Technologies

The paradigm and operationalization of digital health rely on technologies relatively new to healthcare but used in multiple industries over the last several decades. Now emerging into the healthcare ecosystem, they are at the core of the mechanisms of digital health and their impact on and evolution of society. Without new technologies, digital health would not be possible, as they underpin the revolutionary functions of personalized, connected healthcare delivery that permeate the healthcare industry today and into tomorrow.

Defining new technologies, those now emerging into healthcare environments, such as patient care settings, and new models of care such as pay-for-performance, clinical processes and ultimately, the products and solutions of the reality of nurses. Moreover, we also rely on these technologies in our lives daily, for engaging, immersive and ease of experiences for virtual communication, commerce, financial management, education attainment and getting from place to place, to name a few. Termed by Rotolo et al. (2015), new technologies are

> science-based machinery that is characterized by a certain degree of coherence persisting over time and with the potential to employ a considerable impact on the socio-economic domain(s) which is observed in terms of the composition of actors, institutions and patterns of relations among those, along with the concomitant knowledge production processes.

The characteristics of new technologies include radical novelty, fast growth, coherence, noticeable impact and uncertainty and ambiguity.

Core Technologies Impacting Digital Health

Smart automation, wireless, immersive, personalized and connected technologies are all vital to the current functions and advancement of digital health. Individuals are now connected and rely heavily on technology in the dawn of the Fourth Industrial Revolution. This revolution encompasses the development of many disruptive innovations with the characteristics noted previously (Schwab, 2017; Ab Rahman et al., 2017). Permeating healthcare, these emerging technologies include artificial and assistive intelligence (AI), the Internet of Medical Things (IoMT), Virtual and Augmented Reality, genomics and cloud computing. Each impacts digital health in unique ways (Table 2.1). They work together with data to feed the functions of digital health.

The Impact of New Technologies on Digital Health

Digital health products, processes and models, including, but not limited to, smart devices, apps, automation, data storage and provision of virtual care, are fundamental innovations furthering the improvement of health outcomes and advancement of practice in the modern healthcare ecosystem. The significant influence of revolutionary technology is a genuine game changer in the thought processes of care providers of healthcare systems and care providers. The knowledge about how patients access care, understand health status, make care decisions and maintain health through optimized communication and connectedness provides clinician's opportunities for harnessing digital health in a siloed healthcare delivery system.

The massive culture change initiated by using healthcare technologies empowers individuals to be more social in the patient–clinician relationship, autonomous in their care and involved with caregivers to the degree they warrant. Technologies serve as a relative producer and gatekeeper of healthcare data and information, limiting as well as expanding care provision. With these shifts in thought and process, technologies are now more beneficial to end-users and individuals. They collectively inform healthcare quality and safe practices, decrease inefficiencies, waste and care variation and standardize care for improved clinical practice and health outcomes.

Nursing Care Aligning with New Technologies

Healthcare leaders are no longer planning for a future in healthcare where the use of new technologies occurs. Instead, the industry is now immersed

Table 2.1 Examples of New Technologies Impacting Digital Health

New Technology	Definition	Impact on Digital Health
Artificial/Assistive Intelligence (AI)	The automation of smart machines to complete activities that we associate with humans—including thinking, such as decision-making, problem-solving, perceiving, planning and learning and the ability to move objects (Bellman 1978); (Kumar et al. 2018)	• Prediction of events and conditions using Machine Learning • Automation of patient and care staff tasks
Internet of Medical Things (IoMT)	'An amalgamation of medical devices and applications that can connect to healthcare information technology systems using networking technologies.' (Frost & Sullivan 2017)	• Remote patient monitoring • Connected care using sensors
Virtual and Augmented Reality (VR/AR)	'an artificial environment which is experienced through sensory stimuli (such as sights and sounds) provided by a computer and in which one's actions partially determine what happens in the environment' (Merriam-Webster n.d.)	• Management of stressful patient events • Simulation for medical education
Genomics	'The study of all the genes in the human genome together, including their interactions with each other, their environment, and other psychosocial and cultural factors.' (Hamilton 2009)	• Precision health • Personalized health experience
Cloud Computing	'a model which permits ubiquitous, convenient, on-demand network access to a shared pool of configurable computing resources that can be rapidly provisioned and released with minimal management effort or service provider interaction' (Mell & Grance 2011)	• Storage of network healthcare data • Faster patient- care team communications

in the technologies, which are accelerating into patient care and operational settings at a rapid rate. The days where nurses *will* be using these technologies are over. In fact, the time is now to accept the stark realization that emerging technologies that create new care models, processes, products and solutions and significantly impact patient care *are here now*. Nurses using technology will bear the brunt of the implementation of new technologies voluntarily or involuntarily. Nurses can be the purveyors of new technologies adoption and their success in clinical practice and administration.

Twenty-first-century nursing care involves using new technologies to transform how and where nurses deliver patient care and manage operations. Learning new ways of thinking about and processing information using nursing experience, knowledge and skills will transition how nurses work (Robert, 2019). For instance, how nurses receive and review diagnostic information, make clinical decisions, communicate and socialize with patients and their caregivers, and implement nursing interventions with new technologies will augment traditional practices (Barbosa et al., 2021). These new processes will fundamentally change historic nursing care models and enable nurses to provide more holistic, personalized, connected care approaches with new technologies. Further, transformed clinical systems will pivot the focus of nursing care to thinking beyond sickness and acute care to increase focus on new technologies for improving continuity of care across the care continuum, moving patients into the community with intelligent machines and devices and enhancing transitional care with an emphasis on health and wellness.

Health IT Innovation/Disruption Leading to New Technologies

Definition of Health Innovation and Disruption

As we work to understand, support and optimize the digital health ecosystem, it is crucial to comprehend healthcare catalysts for these changes. The terms 'innovation' and 'disruption' are now conventional. Their applications increasingly revolutionize the healthcare industry with the urgent social requirement to shift the make-up of systems and processes. The significant impact innovations have on individuals, clinical care and operations brought forth by the players who are change-makers advancing solutions that improve the health of individuals and populations are quickly becoming the new worldwide standard. Health innovation should be regarded from a global perspective. An exemplary definition comes from the World Health Organization (WHO n.d.):

> Health innovation identifies new or improved health policies, systems, products and technologies, and services and delivery methods that improve people's health and wellbeing. Health innovation responds to unmet public health needs by creating new ways of thinking and working with a focus on the needs of vulnerable populations. It aims to add value in the form of improved efficiency, effectiveness, quality, sustainability, safety and/or affordability. Health innovation can be preventive, promotive, curative and rehabilitative and/or assistive care

(WHO n.d.)

Health innovators, those who aim to change the healthcare industry and meet the imperative of truly working to alter or 'disrupt' antiquated systems in bold and unconventional ways are considered 'disruptors.' These individuals and businesses invent what is next. They shape medicine and develop new ways of ultimately delivering care into the future (Christensen & Hwang, 2007). In general, innovation helps explain the conversion of complicated, expensive products and services into simpler, more affordable ones (Christensen, 2007). In healthcare, this means providing people and populations at all health and socioeconomic statuses to reap the benefits of innovations, including technologies to promote patient-centeredness and enhanced global connectivity and communication.

Current Trends for New Nurse-developed and Nurse-led Technologies for Digital Health: The COVID-19 Pandemic

Nurse innovators are vital to developing, implementing, disseminating and sustaining new technologies in digital health. The COVID-19 pandemic exemplifies this imperative. Since the coronavirus pandemic began, health systems have asked nurses 'to roll up their sleeves' to care for patients using new technologies. Nurses have quickly risen to the occasion to provide personalized digital healthcare for patients and caregivers and promote safe and quality care delivery amid global chaos. Responding to healthcare organizations' call to action during COVID-19 are health IT departments, informatics teams and nurse innovation leaders focusing on digital technologies. Health systems are now addressing emerging challenges to evolve in the new norm. This includes the need for nurses to provide care at a distance. Telehealth visits, remote inpatient consults and family visits, virtual scheduling and the automation of patient triage are key digital health trends. Moreover, the new IT developments of artificial intelligence to allot resources, make clinical decisions and support remote work and communication to keep team members more connected and productive have become commonplace.

These early examples exercised during the pandemic have been successful because they can scale without needing additional resources and can be available at any time and place to patients and caregivers. Dyrda (2020) posits that digital health platforms that enable nurses to orchestrate care between smart machines and humans will make efficiency and being proactive a reality. The technologies that streamline immediate care delivery will no longer be *nice-to-haves* for post-pandemic patients. They will be required for virtual health to grow. To this point, the emerging technology of AI is currently helping patient care teams provide enhanced care. AI-driven tools now afford nurses with differential diagnosis tools that continuously learn with each decision, intelligent chatbots that assist with patient triage, and voice assistants that enable patients to direct and monitor their care in inpatient, ambulatory and virtual settings (Dyrda, 2020).

Nurses have steadily empowered frontline innovators during the pandemic. Now is the time to formalize and systemize their ideas to transform care and digital health (Spader, 2020). The increased need for innovation skills, tools and products, opportunities for learning about innovation and the stark realization that nurses must understand they are natural innovators will have sparked revolutionary digital health services and models during COVID-19. The nurse-led and nurse-developed products that have come to fruition during the coronavirus pandemic will continue to harness innovation. Nurses' gifts of innovation in care delivery will lead them to be the creators, leaders and entrepreneurs of what is next for patients to further the digital health landscape.

Predictive Analytics in Digital Health

Predictive Analytics – A Cornerstone of the Digital Health Model

The purpose of predictive analytics, that is the AI and machine learning (ML) domain, is to predict patterns from historical healthcare data to predict the unknown factors contributing to patient health status and behaviors. Predictive healthcare practice and operations are foundational to most traditional medicine, whether using technology or heuristic methods as approaches to patient care. According to Gandhi and Wang (n.d.), predictive analytics is not reinventing the wheel; it expands how clinicians can practice on a broader and more data-driven scale. The advantage of predictive analytics is being enabled to better measure, aggregate and make sense of the previously hard-to-obtain or non-existent behavioral, psychosocial and biometric data (Gandhi and Wang, n.d.).

One of the key digital health tools to encourage personalized and risk-evasive care delivery is the advanced data analysis models of predictive analytics. With predictive care approaches, it is now possible to track, trend and monitor patients in all physical and virtual care delivery settings and diagnosis, prevent and advance clinical effectiveness through connected and personalized technologies. Using data to predict risk is also paramount to digital health as it anticipates potential problems in real-time to mitigate risks for individuals and whole populations. For instance, patient care teams can now identify at-risk patients in their homes. Forecasting risk prevents emergency care overutilization, hospital readmissions and potential problems. Digital health and wellness tools such as personal medical equipment, intelligent apps, transportation and rehabilitation, support patient services throughout the care continuum including in the community.

Predictive Analytics Primer

Predictive analytics is an AI-driven ML method that uses mathematical and statistical computations to analyze historical data from multiple sources to predict future events. The advanced analytics methodology processes those data, using the ML outputs to gain information to extract the hidden value from newly discovered patterns. It then dynamically informs data-driven decision-making the individuals know, proactively, what will happen, when it will happen and what to do about it (Bari et al., 2017). The purpose of predictive analytics in healthcare is to augment clinicians' clinical decision-making in practice and operations in real-time that impacts clinical care (Sensmeier, 2017). The value of information that predictive analytics imparts is to move from using the two types of data that give hindsight information–descriptive (something happened) and diagnostic (why it happened) data. Instead, harnessing predictive data (when it will happen) and prescriptive data (what we can do about it) enables patient care teams to intervene in clinical care and operational processes proactively before something happens.

With the intent to be assistive in clinical and administrative decision-making, predictive analytics now empowers clinicians to use multi-sourced data-driven technologies, such as sensors, wearables, smart machines and internet-based health portals with more intelligence. Through leveraging these technologies, interventions in clinical and operational situations can become quicker and more accurate, with a higher degree of confidence. This proactivity helps mitigate medical errors, adverse events and near misses and promotes patient health and wellness safely in a more expedited and personalized way.

Real-world Value of Predictive Analytics for Digital Health: Risk-Stratification for Population Management

Today, AI, specifically ML and predictive analytics, processes personalized data, such as demographics, care encounters, medication prescription claims, EHR wearable and sensor data to elicit patient preferences, and help patients and their caregivers participate in the care process. Together, e-health and m-health tools assist patient care teams in using participation to provide high-quality and efficient, personalized care by personalizing 'generic' therapy plans and connecting patients with information beyond those available within their care setting (Shaban-Nejad et al., 2018; Wilk et al., 2017). Focusing on predicting low-risk, rising-risk and high-risk patients is one critical element of population health management. For example, in a virtual medical home setting, prediction helps clinicians stay one step ahead in client care. This type of personalized intervention proves its value by preventing patients from regressing into a need for acute care (Philips, 2020).

During the coronavirus pandemic, a medical home network in the United States (US) reported using ML to identify individuals with a higher risk of developing severe complications from COVID-19. Rather than calling all 122,000 of their members to check in on their wellbeing, the home network took a more targeted, data-driven approach to focus their initial outreach on the 4.4% at-risk patients (Kent, 2020). By educating this group of patients on when and where they should seek medical care, providers sought to proactively help at-risk patients while managing the already strained healthcare system's capacity during the pandemic (Philips, 2020). This approach using predictive analytics pivoted the population health strategy from reactive care delivery to prevention and wellness while gaining efficiencies for the health system.

This example of predictive patient risk stratification for more timely and targeted clinical interventions exemplifies a vital element of digital health—predictive population health management. The digital health strategy mobilized health system data along with robust analytics tools, including critical real-time data-driven reports and dashboard visualizations to strengthen population outcomes for proactive health and wellness. This tracking of population health outcomes fostered anticipated risks to whole populations, such as worsening symptoms, disease progression and progression of chronic illness (Snowdon et al., 2015). In this clinical scenario, the harnessing of predictive and prescriptive data-enabled personalized analytics helped with clinical decision-making by making recommendations to inform holistic, program-level strategies to manage and reduce risks to population segments.

Nursing Current Issues and Considerations for New Technologies

Ethics, Trust and Data Security

Challenges of using new technologies are many despite their growing use in digital health. These include ethics, trust and information security. Because digital health is experiencing fast growth, complications with digital health tools are of great concern at the social and government levels as they can impart human bias, inequity and inaccessibility to individuals, unsolicited sharing of data. These digital health complexities can lead to a lack of adoption by clinicians and patients. Intelligent, automated digital health solutions can introduce human bias as data inputs into the models may include only subsets of populations. Examples of these subsets may include sex and gender, race, social status, geographic locations, and those without access to healthcare (Howard & Borenstein, 2018). For example, doctors heuristically diagnose heart attacks based on symptoms that men experience more commonly than women. Therefore, women are consequently underdiagnosed for heart disease (Rowe, 2021). If this bias exists in the data inputs of automated models that predict and offer suggestions to clinicians, the output that augments decision-making can perpetuate inequality, lead to wrong diagnosis and ineffective treatments and harm equating to low-quality and unsafe patient care delivery. Diversity in data and larger data sets are vital to advance and ensure fairness in using new technology solutions (Kaushal et al., 2020).

Of particular concern is software development companies' technology solutions that use statistical models that feed technologies for predictive analytics, IoMT and genomics. They may have limited transparency to the design and processes. For instance, the automation of AI and specifically ML use algorithms in digital health tools to make recommendations for diagnosis and intervention that exist in a 'black box,' meaning computer models essentially teach themselves to make predictions from large sets of data. Outputs can be questionable due to a lack of interpretability to end-users' use of technologies (Bender, 2019). In addition, personal data and information sharing security are of concern due to the lack of ability to control data's use and maintain privacy for all patients in healthcare and in digital health solutions.

Recommendations for data security and privacy of digital health solutions strategies are beginning to revamp personal data privacy and security laws, such as HIPAA (Health Insurance Portability and Accountability Act of 1996) and GDPR (General Data Protection Regulation). These revised mandates include applying security rules to data users and processors to notify individuals about how they use, store and share data. Consumer requirements for those who process data and use it to develop digital health tools are becoming more stringent (Bari & O'Neill, 2019). There is currently much scrutiny on new technology ethics, fairness and security. Watchdog organizations, government and equity projects specific to upholding justice, software transparency and data security in developing new technologies in digital health are becoming more prominent. The intent of these entities and initiatives exists to ensure technologies used in digital health promote human fairness and safety and encourage principled data practices (Rhee et al., 2019).

Bridging the Consumer Information Gap in Digital Health

Digital health services are changing how individuals manage their health and participate in their care (Smith & Magnani, 2019). With the globally connected nature of digital health, there is a movement to fill the gaps in healthcare consumers' knowledge about using new technologies to empower themselves for proactive personalized health and wellness. Accessibility to use core technologies in digital health is paramount. Health literacy for individuals and populations is needed to bridge the information gap in digital health to leverage it to its fullest extent. The World Health Organization (WHO (n.d.) posits that health literacy is the foundation on which individuals can play an active role in improving their health and engage successfully within communities for optimal health.

In contrast to common health literacy, consumers need to understand more about digital health tools and services beyond everyday tasks of making appointments and reading condition-specific pamphlets. To meet that requirement, advanced knowledge addressing modern digital health literacy is essential. According to Rowlands (n.d.), the emergence of e-health literacy can be a solution. E-health is defined as a healthcare consumer's ability to seek, find, understand and assess health information from electronic sources and apply new knowledge gained to address or solve a health problem.

While digital health is growing exponentially, healthcare consumers lack an understanding of new technologies for better connected and empowered care. Individuals desiring to use data-driven technologies such as telehealth, electronic health records, mobile applications and websites, remote monitoring (Dunn & Hazzard, 2019) cannot acquire the tools needed for digital health. The global reality of a digital divide, the economic and inequalities regarding access to and usage of information and communication technology (Hilfiker et al., 2020), exists as an enormous societal barrier to revolutionary technologies of AI, ML, IoMT and genomics that feed digital health products and services. These barriers exist globally and are largely determined by the geographic location, race, ethnicity, gender and socioeconomic status of individuals seeking healthcare services (Valu, n.d.). Reducing the consumer information gap brought on by social inequalities can focus on improving rural health systems, addressing social determinants of health disparities of individuals in underserved communities and countries, providing them with solutions such as making the foundational tools of digital health, broadband internet and wireless connectivity more readily available (Mullin, 2019). Advancing the understanding and use of technologies and digital health will depend on more global initiatives and government funding to foster the technological connectedness of consumers in the e-health ecosystem and improved health outcomes for those who seek healthcare services using technology.

Digital Health's Impact on Healthcare Consumerism and New Healthcare Models

In our technically connected society, healthcare consumers rely heavily on digital solutions driven by AI, IoMT and cloud computing as they seek healthcare services. These novel technologies will continue to advance as financial, and quality-focused healthcare models evolve from pay-for-volume to pay-for-performance and episodic care bundles, known as value-based care. In the US, new healthcare delivery models are shifting to consumers who demand higher quality and safe healthcare experience—led by the requirements of choice, convenience, transparency, lower cost, personalization with emotional connection and more careful selectivity of health services providers (Heath, 2017). New technologies that fuel digital health tools, models, processes and products can help meet these commanding healthcare consumer criteria.

New technologies are steadily developing to address the rising healthcare costs for consumers. With employers offering high-deductible health plans that pass healthcare costs to employees, consumers can have more consistent engagement in getting the best health service value. According to Vogenberg and Santilli (2018), healthcare consumerism, the transformation of an employer's health benefit plan putting economic purchasing power and decision-making into its members' hands, gives individuals the ability to meet their needs autonomously. Supplying employees with the information and support tools, including those required for digital health, healthcare service providers help support and improve consumers' decisions by offering financial incentives, rewards and other benefits, encouraging personal involvement in altering health and healthcare purchasing behaviors (Vogenberg & Santilli, 2018).

COVID-19 and New Technologies in Digital Health

The COVID-19 is an example of the rapid socialization of global digital health. The coronavirus lockdowns thrust healthcare consumers into the emerging digital health ecosystem, forcing telehealth and virtually delivered care services to keep individuals and healthcare workers safe, remain continuously connected and engaged in their health and wellness. Digital health tools included internet searching for symptoms and diagnosis, intelligent device apps for contact tracing and positive testing surveillance and vaccination site location and verification. The increased use of patient–provider portals that integrate with EHRs has emerged from the pandemic, immersing consumers in being more autonomous out of necessity amid short-staffed and overcrowded hospitals and clinics.

New technologies supporting digital health during the pandemic include AI for predicting the sickest patients for prompt care prioritization, automated chatbots for appointment scheduling and acute care follow-up, and IoT-driven wearables for critical chronic disease management.

Different social media platforms have become foundational for digital health advancement. As dynamic information hubs, social outlets now enable healthcare consumers to get real-time coronavirus statistics and government guidelines and mandates about COVID-related federal and state rules and regulations impacting individuals and communities' public health. Specific tools used by health systems and care providers to support safety and encourage care continuity and commitment to health and wellness during the pandemic have forced healthcare consumers to be more hands-on and proactive and preventative about their health. As the pandemic continues, new and better healthcare services and products will advance digital healthcare delivery and payment models for consumers into more technological-driven routines and health service procurement and clinical practices for healthcare providers?

Operationalizing New Technologies for Digital Health

Nurse and IT Expert Partnerships for Development and Implementation

To sustain healthcare innovation at an economically and fiscally responsible pace, a collaborative effort requiring input from diverse stakeholders and key players in the industry is vital. With the continued global applications of digital technologies, the rapid expansion of digital health occurs through divergent collaboration among global leaders of digital innovation in the healthcare industry.

The partnership between key players in both the private and public sectors and academia has engineered a growing list of innovative digital healthcare solutions (Pando, 2017). Divergent collaborations in the technology space are ones that emerge from innovation collectives. Healthcare organizations are actively working together with big IT companies, startups and academic institutions to solve healthcare business problems. Born from these partnerships are new technology solutions which are cataloged and disseminated to create new businesses and innovation centers in healthcare systems, organizations and institutes (Figure 2.1) (Carroll, 2021).

Nurses are vital stakeholders in divergent collaborations for digital health. In the process of divergent collaborations, nurses must be front and center to partner with vendors and institutions to conceptualize, develop, test, implement, market and sustain digital health technologies. Nurses must

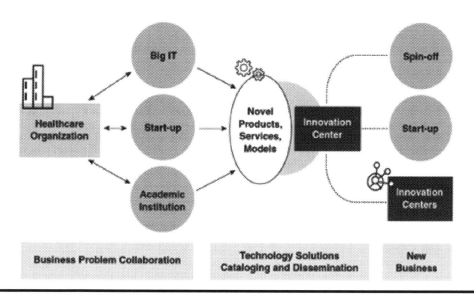

Figure 2.1   Model for new technology centers.

advance policy that defines and regulates the application and implications of new technologies. There is currently a shift in the digital health ecosystem to welcome the nursing perspective, including their skills, knowledge and innovative spirit into the divergent collaboration process. Roles include executive leadership and contributors on project teams, with a growing trend of nurses actively participating in digital healthcare IT tools' digital strategy and research and development.

Interoperability—Harmonizing the Siloes of Data and Information for Digital Health

Digital health tools, models, processes and products that promote healthcare consumer connectedness depend on *Interoperability*, the ability of two or more systems or components to exchange information and use the information exchanged (Lehne et al., 2019). There are different sub-definitions of interoperability components, layers or levels including a distinction between lower-level technical components and higher-level organizational components. According to Snowden (2020), four components of digital health operationalization and interoperability are essential. The first is *Foundational*, the exchange of data accessible across clinical settings. The next is *Organizational*, the use of governance tools such as policy, security and privacy. The third is *Semantic*: the enablement of analytics tools and reporting to streamline data access and management. And the fourth is

Structural: data centralization, automation and integration for seamless data flow (Snowden, 2020).

Making disparate healthcare data sources and repositories interoperable has been a challenge. However, interoperability is vital to operationalize new technologies core to digital health. Connecting data sources for successful use in new technologies include Application Programming Interfaces (APIs), as they are communication points between systems. With APIs, healthcare IT developers are simplifying interoperability to provide healthcare professionals and users' data more efficiently (O'Dowd n.d.). APIs are pieces of code that expose data from underlying information systems in industry-standard formats, including FHIR (Fast Healthcare Interoperability Resources) specification, along with the now-common use of HL7 v2. APIs enable uniform, scalable and repeatable integrations that accelerate development cycles through standardization and reuse (Padmanabhan, 2020). The dependence on data sharing to use new technologies in digital health, such as AI and IoMT, enabled by APIs, will forge a way for health systems, providers, payers and patient care teams to connect siloed technology systems and digital health sources of data. It is necessary to realize the use and value of predictive analytics to further proactive, personalized risk-focused care to track, trend and trace health outcomes across the patient care journey of care to identify risk and develop strategies for care quality and safety (Snowden, 2020).

New Skills and Roles for Nurses and in the Age of Digital Health

The success of digital health is dependent on nurses' understanding, adoption and application of new technologies in clinical practice in all settings, from the hospital to ambulatory settings and into the community. To stay relevant in the ever-evolving digital health landscape, nurses must use their current clinical skills and knowledge and gain new skills to use digital health's foundational new intelligent, connected and personalized AI, IoMT, cloud computing technologies and genomics. For example, beyond using the current iteration of EHRs, nurse leaders recommend that globally connected care requires nurses to gain new skills and mindset about new technologies and be ready for next-generation EHRs that incorporate AI (Luppa, 2020).

With the advancement of digital health, new opportunities are coming for nurses in all specialties, including informatics. Opportunities to use them to establish population health models that are functional and sustainable are clear. New roles will emerge, including nurse navigators, disease managers, care advocates and wellness coaches enhanced by including new technology. This will allow nurses to transform care delivery for healthcare consumers. Nurses' primary goal will be to train people and populations to use and adapt to new digital health tools, models and services to support improved health literacy, access aspects of the digital divide and encourage them to be more proactive and empowered in their health and wellness.

Conclusion

The worldwide culture change initiated by using new healthcare technologies empowers individuals to be more social in the patient–clinician relationship, which are proactive, empowered, and autonomous in their care and seeking healthcare services. Nurses can now harness new technologies for digital health—continuity of care, moving patients into the community with intelligent machines and devices, enhancing transitional care and flow along their journey throughout the care continuum with an emphasis on personalized and engaging health and wellness. Nurse-led and developed innovation has been evident during the COVID-19 pandemic. Now is the time to formalize and implement these ideas to transform care and advance digital health. With the intent to be assistive in clinical and administrative decision-making, particularly in digital health, predictive analytics now empowers decision-makers to use multi-sourced data-driven technologies. These include data from sensors, wearables, smart machines and internet-based health portals. Data and information must be interoperable, scalable and free of bias to promote safety and equity for consumers. With the global socialization of digital health, there is a movement promoting health literacy, as consumers need to understand technology-driven tools and services beyond everyday tasks. Both patient and nurses' advanced knowledge addressing modern digital health literacy is essential to meet that requirement. The future will require nurses to partner with health information technology experts to lend the nursing perspective to new models, processes, services, and products, and stay relevant in the ever-evolving digital health landscape by applying their current clinical skills and knowledge and gain new skills to advance global digital health in the 21st century.

References

Ab Rahman, A., Abdul Hamid, U. K., & Chin, T. A. (2017). Emerging technologies with disruptive effects: A review. *PERINTIS eJournal*, 7(2), pp.111–128 [online]. Available at: https://perintis.org.my/ejournal/wp-content/uploads/2018/11/Paper-4-Vol.-7-No.-2-pp.-111-128.pdf (Accessed 25 April 2021).

Bari A., Chaouchi, M., & Jung, T. (2017). *Predictive analytics for dummies.* 2nd ed. Hoboken, NJ: Wiley.

Bari, L., & O'Neill, D. (2019). Rethinking patient data privacy in the era of digital health. *Health Affairs* [online]. Available at: https://www.healthaffairs.org/do/10.1377/hblog20191210.216658/full/ (Accessed 26 December 2021).

Bellman, R. E. (1978). *An introduction to artificial intelligence: Can computers think?* San Francisco, CA: Boyd & Fraser Publishing.

Bender, E. (2019). *Unpacking the black box in artificial intelligence for medicine.* [online]. Available at: https://undark.org/2019/12/04/black-box-artificial-intelligence (Accessed 27 May 2021).

Carroll, W. M., ed. (2021). *Emerging technologies for nurses: Implications for practice.* 1st ed. New York: Springer Publishing Company.

Christensen, C. M. (2007). *The innovator's dilemma: When new technologies cause great firms to fail.* Boston, MA: Harvard Business School Press.

Christensen, C. M., & Hwang, J. (2007). Perspective: Innovation–disruptive innovation in health care delivery: A framework for business-model innovation. *Health Affairs*, 27(5), pp.1329–1335.

Dunn, P., & Hazzard, E. (2019). Technology approaches to digital health literacy. *International Journal of Cardiology*, 293, pp.294–296. https://doi.org/10.1016/j.ijcard.2019.06.039

Dyrda, L. (2020). COVID-19 innovations will outlive pandemic. *Becker's Hospital Review* [online]. Available at: https://www.beckershospitalreview.com/digital-transformation/the-legacy-of-covid-19-how-key-innovations-will-outlive-the-pandemic.html (Accessed 2 May 2021).

Frost & Sullivan. (2017). *Internet of medical things revolutionizing healthcare* [online]. Available at: https://aabme.asme.org/posts/internet-of-medical-things-revolutionizing-healthcare (Accessed 25 April 2021).

Gandhi, M., & Wang, T. (n.d.). *The future of personalized healthcare: Predictive analytics* [online]. Available at: https://rockhealth.com/reports/predictive-analytics/ (Accessed 22 May 2021).

Hamilton, R. (2009). Nursing advocacy in a postgenomic age. *Nursing Clinics of North America*, 44(4), pp.435–446.

Heath, S. (2017). *Retail consumer experience key in consumer-driven healthcare* [online]. Available at: https://patientengagementhit.com/news/retail-consumer-experience-key-in-consumer-driven-healthcare (Accessed 30 May 2021).

Howard, A. & Borenstein, J. (2018). The ugly truth about ourselves and our robot creations: The problem of bias and social inequity. *Science and Engineering Ethics*, 24, pp.1521–1536. https://doi.org/10.1007/s11948-017-9975-2

Hilfiker, S. W., Santana, S., Freedman, M., & Harris, L. M. (2020). There's a gap between digital health information and users: Let's close it. *Studies in Health Technology and Informatics*, 269, pp.324–331. https://doi.org/10.3233/SHTI200047

Kaushal, A., Altman, R., & Langlotz, C. (2020). Health care AI systems are biased. *Scientific American* [online]. Available at: https://www.scientificamerican.com/article/health-care-ai-systems-are-biased/ (Accessed 27 May 2021).

Kent, J. (2020). *Leveraging AI for COVID-19 outreach, population health management.* HealthITAnalytics [online]. Available at: https://healthitanalytics.com/news/leveraging-ai-for-covid-19-outreach-population-health-management (Accessed 23 May 2021).

Kumar, A., Shukla, P., Sharan, A. & Mahindru, T. (2018). *National strategy for artificial intelligence* [online]. Available at: http://niti.gov.in/writereaddata/fi les/d ocument_publication/NationalStrategy-for-AI-Discussion-Paper.pdf (Accessed 25 April 2021).

Lehne, M., Sass, J., Essenwanger, A., Schepers, J., & Thun, S. (2019). Why digital medicine depends on interoperability. *NPJ Digital Medicine,* 2(79) [online]. Available at: https://doi.org/10.1038/s41746-019-0158-1 (Accessed 26 December 2021).

Luppa, N. (2020). *Let's get digital: Nursing in a digital world preparing for digital nursing practice* [online]. Available at https://consultqd.clevelandclinic.org/lets-get-digital-nursing-in-a-digital-world/ (Accessed 30 May 2021).

Mell, P., & Grance, T. (2011). *The NIST definition of cloud computing* [online]. Available at: http://faculty.winthrop.edu/domanm/csci411/Handouts/NIST.pdf (Accessed 25 April 2021).

Merriam-Webster (n.d.) *Virtual reality | definition of virtual reality* [online]. Available at: https://www.merriam-webster.com/dictionary/virtual%20reality (Accessed 25 April 2021).

Mullin, R. (2019). *Bridging the digital divide: Expanding internet and rural healthcare access* [online]. Available at: https://www.healthitanswers.net/bridging-the-digital-divide-expanding-internet-and-rural-healthcare-access/ (Accessed 28 May 2021).

O'Dowd, E. (n.d.). *Why application programming interfaces are key for healthcare.* [online]. Available at: https://hitinfrastructure.com/features/why-application-programming-interfaces-are-key-for-healthcare (Accessed 31 May 2021).

Padmanabhan, P. (2020). *Why interoperability is cool (again)* [online]. Available at: https://www.healthcareitnews.com/blog/why-interoperability-cool-again (Accessed 30 May 2021).

Pando, A. (2017). Collaborative innovation is necessary to advance in health care. *Forbes Magazine* [online]. Available at: https://www.forbes.com/sites/forbestechcouncil/2017/09/19/collaborative-innovation-is-necessary-to-advance-in-health-care (Accessed 2 May 2021).

Philips (2020). *Predictive analytics in healthcare: Three real-world examples.* Philips [online]. Available at: https://www.philips.com/a-w/about/news/archive/featu res/20200604-predictive-analytics-in-healthcare-three-real-world-examples.html (Accessed 22 May 2021).

Rhee, et al. (2019). *AI now 2019 report.* AI Now Institute [online]. Available at: https://ainowinstitute.org/AI_Now_2019_Report.html (Accessed 27 May 2021).

Robert, N. (2019). How artificial intelligence is changing nursing. *Nursing Management,* 50(9), pp.30–39.

Rotolo, D., Hicks, D., & Martin, B. R. (2015). What is an emerging technology? *Research Policy,* 44(10), pp.1827–1843.

Rowe, J. (2021). *Wanted: 'AI algorithms without bias'* [online]. Available at: https://www.healthcareitnews.com/ai-powered-healthcare/wanted-ai-algorithms-without-bias (Accessed 27 May 2021).

Rowlands, G. (n.d.). *Digital health literacy* [online]. Available at: https://www.who.int/global-coordination-mechanism/activities/working-groups/17-s5-rowlands.pdf (Accessed 28 May 2021).

Schwab, K. (2017). *The fourth industrial revolution*. New York: Crown Publishing Group.

Sensmeier, J. (2017). Harnessing the power of artificial intelligence. *Nursing Management*, 48(11), pp.14–19.

Shaban-Nejad, A., Michalowski, M., & Buckeridge, D. L. (2018). Health intelligence: How artificial intelligence transforms population and personalized health. *NPJ Digital Medicine*, 1(53), pp.1–2. https://doi.org/10.1038/s41746-018-0058-9

Smith, B., & Magnani, J. W. (2019). New technologies, new disparities: The intersection of electronic health and digital health literacy. *International Journal of Cardiology*, 292, pp.280–282. https://doi.org/10.1016/j.ijcard.2019.05.066

Snowden, A. W. (2020). Advancing digital health transformation: The HIMSS digital health indicator. *Healthcare Information Management and Systems Society* [webinar slides].

Snowdon, A. W., Alessi, C., Bassi, H., DeForge, R. T., & Schnarr, K. (2015). Enhancing patient experience through personalization of health services. *Healthcare Management Forum*, 28(5), pp.182–185.

Spader, C. (2020). *The new normal: Nurses as innovators*. My American Nurse [online]. Available at: https://www.myamericannurse.com/the-new-normal-nurses-as-innovators/ (Accessed 8 May 2021).

Valu, M. (n.d.). *Understanding the digital divide and ensuring access for all* [online]. Available at: https://www.himss.org/resources/understanding-digital-divide-and-ensuring-access-all (Accessed 28 May 2021).

Vogenberg, F. R., & Santilli, J. (2018). Industry trends: Healthcare trends for 2018. *American Health and Drug Benefits*, 11(1), pp.48–54.

Wilk, S. et al. (2017). Comprehensive mitigation framework for concurrent application of multiple clinical practice guidelines. *Journal of Biomedical Informatics*, 66, pp.52–71.

World Health Organization (WHO). (n.d.a). *Health promotion: Health literacy* [online]. Available at: https://www.who.int/healthpromotion/health-literacy/en/ (Accessed 28 May 2021).

WHO. (n.d.b). *Health topics–innovation* [online]. Available at: https://www.who.int/topics/innovation/en/ (Accessed 2 May 2021).

Chapter 3

Opportunities and Challenges for Digital Health Advancement

Gillian Strudwick, Sanaz Riahi and Nicholas R. Hardiker

Contents

Introduction

Throughout the last few decades, there has been a consistent discussion about how the healthcare field will significantly transform given the digital advances present in most people's everyday lives. Some examples of these digital advancements include the use of automated voice assistants, new

DOI: 10.4324/9781003054849-3

forms of social media, computers in our pockets (smartphones), remote home monitoring and beyond. These forms of technology have become ubiquitous for numerous individuals around the world, and many people rely on these technologies to perform their day-to-day activities. For example, rides can be booked via a mobile app, hair appointments and food delivery booked online, home heating and monitoring controlled remotely, alarms activated by voice commands and the list goes on. It is not hard to imagine why individuals may want and expect that the digital technologies that they utilize in their everyday lives should also be available within the healthcare domain. These digital technologies have allowed for numerous conveniences in other sectors, so it may be expected that these same conveniences are present in healthcare.

To date, however, there is often a gap between the wishes and expectations of those seeking health services and the realities of the current environment (Booth, 2016). The healthcare environment is yet to have a radical transformation in terms of the ubiquitous use of digital technologies comparable to that of those used in the non-healthcare sector. A number of barriers unique to the health domain have made it challenging to advance digital health in similar ways that we use technology in our personal lives. These may be related to the knowledge and skill of health professionals in knowing about and using the digital technologies available to them (Booth, 2006; Risling, 2017), our ability to use digital technologies in compassionate ways (Kemp et al., 2020), the need to empower patients in using digital technologies (Ammenwerth et al., 2019), data silos and issues of interoperability, the need for open science/data, digital health equity and beyond. This chapter will explore these key issues with the purpose of providing an overview of the various opportunities for digital health advancement that exist and providing strategies and solutions to the current challenges preventing this advancement from being fully realized.

Opportunities for Digital Health Advancements

Numerous opportunities for digital health advancement exist by leveraging some of the physical technologies and lessons learned from those used in our personal lives to the healthcare context. The following section of this chapter will review areas that are ripe for digital health advancement, while describing some of the key challenges that have existed to date in doing so.

Digital Compassion

Digital compassion is a relatively new concept for many, although the idea of digital compassion is essentially an extension of the compassionate care we strive to deliver in healthcare environments, however in this case in digital forms (Wiljer et al., 2019). While the feeling of empathy is often understood as "walking in someone's shoes" as a way of obtaining a feeling of understanding what an individual is going through, compassion is an extension beyond empathy in that it involves a response or action. Thus, compassion is both about trying to understand what someone is going through and then acting in a way to address or alleviate pain, suffering or an undesirable state. Digital technologies may be used to both help understand what someone else is going through, and to support an action that is aimed at alleviating some or all of the burden (Kemp et al., 2020). As digital technologies become increasingly more present, there may be a fear that the human and compassionate side of healthcare is being reduced or eliminated, with efficiency and the need for 'data' taking a central spot.

While the benefits of providing digital compassion can be likely understood, several barriers are present that likely serve as preventing digital compassion from being fully enacted in our healthcare environments. First, many healthcare professionals have received little formal training with regards to digital health and informatics in their entry-to-practice programs, and since the concept of digital compassion is somewhat new, it is likely that healthcare professionals haven't received any education or training on this specific topic. Second, many organizations in which healthcare professionals practice are in the midst of creating environments in which this digital compassion can take place. That said, existing structures (e.g. older buildings not equipped to support modern-day healthcare delivery) and lack of knowledge from leadership may hinder the supports required for digital compassion to be present. Finally, the features of technology that allow them to be used in compassionate ways are not yet fully understood, and thus this area is one that could see significant growth in the coming decades.

Health Professional Competencies

An interaction with the healthcare system most often involves working with, communicating or receiving care from healthcare professionals. To advance care through digital technologies, these healthcare professionals need to be aware of the digital technologies that exist and can be used in care delivery, as well as how best to use these technologies to maximize both the experience of individuals receiving care and their outcomes. Essentially, healthcare professionals need to hold competencies relevant to the digital health and informatics field to be able to deliver care in a sufficient way in a technological world (Staggers et al., 2001). To date, some healthcare professional groups receive digital health and informatics-specific content in their entry-to-practice level education. This seems to vary by profession and by country and is a relatively recent addition to these programs, meaning that the majority of healthcare professionals practicing in today's clinical environments have not had this requisite education and may not have developed these competencies in their workplaces. In addition, those working in leadership roles, which often occur at a later career stage, have in many cases not obtained the requisite technological competencies to be effective in advancing care through digital technologies (Strudwick et al., 2019). Thus, this provides a challenge for how digital technologies can be best selected, implemented, evaluated and used in clinical contexts today.

Patient Empowerment

Patient empowerment is seen as a core value of high-quality patient-centered care (Health Organization and Office for Europe, 2013; Bonsignore et al., 2015). The idea of advancing patient empowerment with digital health tools to achieve better health outcomes is a vision that has many proponents in healthcare. However, this vision to transform healthcare has not been realized entirely (Morley & Floridi, 2020).

The concept of 'empowerment' is rooted in the social action and civil rights movement during the 1960s and has also been present in the literature in a diverse range of fields (Pekonen et al., 2020; Morley & Floridi, 2020). Although the concept has been around in healthcare since the 1980s, more specifically in patients' care and education in chronic conditions (Pekonen et al., 2020), there has been a renewed interest in more recent years with the increased presence of technology and consumer demand (Cerezo et al., 2016). Publications on patient empowerment have also become more increasingly present within the digital health literature, with an emerging theme that the future of patient empowerment has great possibilities as a result of technological advancements and better access of patients to these technologies (Kambhampati et al., 2016). However, there is also a lack of clear linkage between the use of digital health services, patient empowerment and health outcomes in a pervasive manner. Certainly, there are studies that have demonstrated that patient empowerment is related to better health outcomes, such as well-being, self-management (Chen & Li, 2009; Londoño & Schulz, 2015), health status (Jerofke et al., 2014), health-related quality of life (Koekenbier et al., 2016) and cost-effectiveness (Bergman - Chalmers, 2014). However, these types of outcomes related to patient empowerment are not ubiquitous in healthcare as a result of not being measured and or operationalized effectively and consistently.

One challenge that contributes to the suboptimal achievement of this vision is the lack of consensus and clarity on the definition and operationalization of patient empowerment (Risling et al., 2017; Barr et al., 2015; Morley & Floridi, 2020). One example of a definition is provided by the World Health Organization, describing empowerment as 'a process through which people gain greater control over decisions and actions affecting their health' (Health Promotion Glossary, 1998). Another existing challenge is the gaps and inconsistencies in how empowerment is measured. A recent systematic review identifying generic instruments to measure patient empowerment only reported three instruments which measured empowerment most comprehensively with evidence of acceptable validity and reliability (Pekonen et al., 2020). The review also highlighted the reality that the majority of the instruments developed in this domain have been only in the last ten years, which explains the current challenge.

The idea of empowering people with digital health tools to take better care of their health is very appealing and one that is worth efforts to continue striving to achieve. There is a need to begin with understanding what empowerment actually means and develop a more complex critical analysis of the ways in which it can be operationalized by levering digital health strategies. Indeed, currently in healthcare, there are many promising evidences that enabling patient empowerment has the potential for many positive outcomes. The challenges and the opportunities are eliminating the current discords in definition, operationalization strategies and measurement to aid in greater universal presence and success of patient empowerment in healthcare.

Data Sharing

The digitization of healthcare has been advancing over the last decade. This in turn has generated a steep rise in the production of health data that comes not only from health systems (healthcare records, MRI scanners, clinical test data, etc.) but also from wearable devices. All of these data combined form 'big data' that have great promise for improving health systems, as well as individual care (Hulsen et al., 2019). The idea of patient data sharing to enable scientific progress is gaining much momentum, mostly as a result of the power of big data analysis, machine learning, artificial intelligence, etc. Furthermore, big data can provide insight and predictions into causes of diseases and effects of treatment, while also facilitating analysis tailored to an individual's characteristics (personalized medicine). However, when discussing sharing of patient data, there is a lack of consensus on who actually owns the data (Kostkova et al., 2016). Health institutions tend to believe that they own the patient data because they are the ones collecting them, though they are, in fact, the 'data custodians.' The data is actually the property of the patient, and the access and use of the data outside of the clinical setting usually requires patient consent (Hulsen et al., 2019). This data ownership becomes even more vague in relation to real-time big data streams generated by social media and increasingly popular tracking/wearable devices.

As a result of all of this, there is an increasingly urgent need to balance the opportunities created by big data to improve healthcare against the rights of individuals. Specifically, the major concerns are related to privacy, confidentiality, data ethics and control over data about individuals once it is shared. These concerns are consequences of an absence of transparent data ownership regulation, resulting in varying approaches toward data ownership, usage and responsibility related to sharing and accountability (Olson, 2014; Hulsen et al., 2019).

While health systems that have taken the lead in using big data and its analysis have demonstrated significant benefits in clinical and administrative functions, barriers related to transparent regulations have limited the opportunities toward health system transformation and advancements in personalized medicine. Policies and regulations at local, national and international levels are necessary to standardize practices and enable data sharing and access, while equally ensuring data ethics, protecting individuals' privacy, confidentiality and control.

Digital Health Equity

The response to the COVID-19 pandemic has required an accelerated adoption of digital health solutions to ensure ongoing access to clinical care and enable adherence to public health measures in mitigating the transmission and spread of the virus. However, these recent events have further exacerbated the long-existing inequities of access to and implementation of digital health, as well as the quality of care afforded by digital health (Crawford & Serhal, 2020). In the development of digital health solutions, generally, there has been a lack of attention to health equity (Sinha & Schryer-Roy, 2018). With the proliferation of digital solutions in response to the pandemic, there have been unintended consequences of furthering health inequities. Having limited or lack of access to technology due to such factors as poverty, under-resourcing of health systems and neighborhoods, and homelessness contribute to the current digital health inequities. Other factors that need to be considered for digital health technologies are the social, cultural and economic realities, as well as social determinants of health, which all directly and or indirectly impact health equity (Were et al., 2019; Crawford & Serhal, 2020).

There are multiple opportunities toward creating a more equitable technology landscape. One strategy is for measuring and increasing broadband access at the local and national levels. Health professionals need to also include assessing for technology access as part of their standard of care, which enables health institutions to understand and influence the digital health inequities being experienced by their patients. Another strategy includes digital health technologies consistently including sociodemographic and digital literacy metrics as part of their implementation plans (Rodriguez et al., 2020). Technology companies need to adopt improved patient-centric designs with greater inclusion of diverse patient populations. Lastly, ensuring there are policies, standards and guidelines that mandate digital health equity.

Nursing Records

There is evidence to indicate that certain components of Electronic Health Records (EHR) can support improvements in nursing practice. For example, well-designed systems that are integrated into the clinical workflow can support communication (Motamedi et al., 2011) and handover (Starmer et al., 2013). However, an ongoing issue for EHR systems is that they were largely developed independently of workflow and without the input of nurses and other end-users (Kossman et al., 2013; Rogers et al., 2013; Yu et al., 2013).

Almost all existing EHR systems have been developed using an approach to the documentation of healthcare that has been adapted from the 'written' world; normally consisting of modules such as computerized physician order entry (CPOE), medication prescribing and administration, doctors notes,

nursing notes and other elements (such as laboratory reporting and computerized decision support). As a consequence, users of EHR systems highlight
a range of problems, such as poor fit with workflow, which requires users to
develop 'workarounds' (Dowding et al., 2014).

While other studies may have considered specific structural and functional aspects of nursing records (Saranto et al., 2014), one of the most recent
attempts to evaluate the impact of different nursing records systems systematically was the Cochrane Library systematic review 'Nursing Record Systems:
effects of nursing practice and healthcare outcomes' (Urquhart et al., 2009).

Under the Cochrane review, a nursing record system is described as 'the
record of care that is planned or given to individual patients and clients by
qualified nurses or by other caregivers (including nursing students) under
the direction of a qualified nurse' (p. 3); under this description, a nursing record can clearly take different forms. The review explored a range of
bibliographic sources and identified from a comprehensive search strategy a
large number (over 6,300) of potentially relevant articles. However, only nine
articles were considered eligible for inclusion (i.e., in scope and of sufficient
rigor). And while some of the studies demonstrated that individual nursing
record systems might provide solutions to specific problems, such as miss-
ing notes, it is unclear the difference that any change in the nursing record
system actually makes in terms of practice or outcomes. This indicates, to
some extent, a lack of understanding of the benefits of individual nursing
record systems themselves. An earlier review (Urquhart & Currell, 2005) had
also concluded that nursing records do not actually reflect nursing practice.
Although there had been plans for a further update, the Cochrane review
was subsequently discontinued, partly due to the lack of significant additional evidence between revision cycles.

The issues highlighted above, coupled with the realization that existing
nursing record systems may not be able to reveal their intended benefits,
brings into question the architecture or foundations upon which nursing
documentation is built and suggests a need for a re-interpretation by nursing
itself of the nursing record, purposefully framed within an electronic context, including a new agreed specification for a novel approach that fits with
workflow and meets the information needs of nursing.

Terminologies for Nursing

Over the last half-century, a number of factors may have conspired to
drive or support the development of standardized languages or agreed on

terminologies to support nursing practice. These range from the profession-alization of nursing (Keogh, 1997) and the desire to make visible its unique contribution to healthcare, to the adoption within healthcare of electronic health records and the possibilities that this offered around enhanced data management (Rutherford, 2008). Early enthusiasm among nurse schol-ars gave rise to a number of standardized terminologies that were widely reported and recognized by a number of bodies at the time of their devel-opment and initial adoption. Many of these terminologies remain in use in education and/or in practice today (Standardized nursing languages: essential for the nursing workforce. n.d.).

While there is a degree of overlap between these terminologies, unsur-prisingly perhaps in terms of content, there are also differences in structure, style and intended scope. Each terminology exhibits its own balance of interface characteristics (relating to the role of terminologies in data capture and presentation) and reference characteristics (related to the role of ter-minologies in data aggregation and analysis and interoperability between systems) (Ziebarth, 2018). Related to these role-based characteristics, each terminology is set within its own organizing structure, and each terminology also exhibits its own balance of enumeration and composition.

The terminologies that emerged in the formative years tend toward simple lists, often set within their own theoretical framework, for example, NANDA (Rutherford, 2008; Ziebarth, 2018), and accompanied by their own proposed recording structure/process, for example, The Omaha System (Garvin et al., 2008). Certain of these longer-standing terminologies also display a modest degree of selective compositionality to support post-coordination of related entities, for example, Clinical Care Classification (CCC) (Arnold et al., 2007). Without a doubt, these terminologies have helped the profession to scope out, and to a degree to bound, nurse recording practice. They may have also helped to make nursing more visible within EHRs. However, and perhaps with notable exceptions, these early terminologies have not delivered fully on the promise of more data-enabled or data-driven nursing practice.

Nurse researchers were quick to recognize the potential of more con-temporary approaches to terminology development. The International Classification for Nursing Practice (ICNP) (Coenen, 2003), a product of the International Council of Nurses, was perhaps the first terminology for nurs-ing to deploy description logic in its development. Description logics are formal knowledge representation languages that are used to describe and reason on concepts or entities within a particular domain (Meditskos et al., 2017), in this case, nursing practice. Since its first release version, ICNP has been underpinned by the *de facto* description logic standard, Web Ontology Language (OWL). A similar approach has been taken more recently by Systematized Nomenclature of Human and Veterinary Medicine SNOMED International, to support the development of SNOMED Clinical Terms CT (SNOMED CT, 2020), a more comprehensive multidisciplinary terminology for health and social care (the World Health Organization (WHO), has also deployed OWL to support the development of the foundation for the 11th revision of the International Classification of Diseases (ICD 11) (ICD-11, 2019)).

The parallel development of a range of nursing terminologies has provided nurse users with a degree of choice over which particular terminology to use to record their practice, and this may be serving to ensure a good fit with particular settings and cultures. However, the differences between this range of terminologies, coupled with poor interoperability between individual terminologies, may be serving also to fragment the nursing information space, thereby preventing nursing from leveraging the potential of information to advance the profession.

Many people have been working for many years to ensure that nursing is faithfully represented in EHRs. However, the terminologies that have been developed to support nursing recording practice either have been based on tradition or represent little more than our 'best guess' at what might be useful. The result of the practical application, over many years, of a multiplicity of nursing terminologies, is a highly fragmented global nursing data repository. Now, with the emergence of contemporary data science, nursing needs a higher degree of data harmonization, so that it can begin to determine what data it really needs to transform and advance the profession and to improve the health of citizens worldwide.

In order to facilitate the harmonization of nursing data, building on previous mapping work of the International Council of Nursing (ICN) and SNOMED International entered into an agreement in 2020 to work toward integrating ICNP into SNOMED CT (with the two organizations retaining ownership and control of their respective terminologies) (ICN and SNOMED sign ground-breaking agreement to secure a bright future for the International Classification for Nursing Practice, 2021). While this does not rule out the continued use of other nursing terminologies, the hope is that with increased uptake and use, the profession can move more determinedly toward more consistent nursing data collection and a greater understanding of what data is needed and how it might be used to support nursing.

Artificial Intelligence

Although engagement of nurses with Artificial Intelligence (AI) is not widespread, and understanding across the profession may be limited, there are notable examples of how the application of AI methods and techniques can support nursing and potentially improve health (Clancy, 2020), including data mining to identify falls risk (Topaz et al., 2019) and machine learning to support coding from the nursing text (Moen et al., 2020).

The development and application of intelligent software have the potential to enhance nursing care by relieving nurses of routine activities and releasing time for direct patient care. However, AI might also introduce unintended (or intended) negative consequences, such as the reinforcement of bias in decision support (Obermeyer et al., 2019) (regarding this example, note that with prudent development and implementation, AI is as likely to help identify bias and therefore enhance decision making (Silberg & Manyika, 2019)). Thus, it is important that nurses are involved centrally in scoping out possibilities for AI (Pepito & Locsin, 2019).

While nurses may share the long-standing anxiety of people being replaced by intelligent machines (made manifest by the Turing Test or 'imitation game') (Turing, 1950), a number of scholars have argued the ongoing need for a degree of clinical interpretation and evaluation to address uncertainties introduced by AI, for example in AI-based decision support (Shortliffe & Sepúlveda, 2018; Eisenhauer et al., 2007). This obviously points to a need for a degree of understanding of AI and its capabilities and limitations (Davenport & Kalakota, 2019), as articulated for other contexts (McGrow, 2019), which in turn requires the engagement of nurses as collaborators in development (Matinolli et al., 2020).

A number of nursing scholars have argued for a greater understanding of AI across the profession, the involvement of nurses in AI development and implementation, and engagement of the profession with the underlying morals and applied ethics of AI (Ronquillo et al., 2021). The proactive engagement of the profession with AI can only enhance the resulting technologies, for nursing, for other professional groups and critically for citizens.

Forecasting the Future

In looking ahead to the immediate future, there is likely to be an increasing digitization of health services and data-informed healthcare. This will include significant energy, time and resources aimed at addressing the identified challenges discussed in this chapter that prevent the realization of many digital technology benefits from being realized. Long term, as proficiency in managing these common challenges improves, there may be a shift in that the digital technology efficiencies and conveniences that are achieved in non-healthcare contexts are more easily converted into the health space. This likely includes increased reliance on automation, artificial intelligence (e.g. decisions assisted via machine learning), chatbots, robots and beyond.

Conclusion

This chapter provided an overview of some of the opportunities that exist currently to advance the digital health agenda for nursing. These opportunities span the areas of digital compassion, health professional competencies, patient empowerment, data sharing, digital health equity, nursing records, terminologies for nursing, artificial intelligence and beyond. Challenges, however, exist in being able to fully realize the potential of digital technologies in the health context as they relate to the opportunities brought forward. These extend beyond the nursing profession and into the broader digital health community. Given the gap between the digital technologies that are used in the everyday lives of individuals, there is a need to address these gaps in a timeline and coordinated manner. Without doing so, we run the risk of healthcare environments falling short in meeting the expectations and needs of people requiring care.

References

Ammenwerth, E., Hoerbst, A., Lannig, S., Mueller, G., Siebert, U., & Schnell-Inderst, P. (2019). Effects of adult patient portals on patient empowerment and health-related outcomes: A systematic review. *MEDINFO 2019: Health and Wellbeing e-Networks for All*, pp.1106–1110. https://doi.org/10.3233/SHTI190397

Arnold, J., Bakken, S., Feeg, V., Holzemer, W., Huff, S., Konicek, D., Lee, N., Matney, S., McCormick, K., & Taylor, S. (2007). *Clinical care classification (CCC) system manual: A guide to nursing: Virginia Saba, EdD, RN, FAAN: Google books*. New York: Springer Publishing Company.

Barr, P. J., Scholl, I., Bravo, P., Faber, M. J., Elwyn, G., & McAllister, M. (2015). Assessment of patient empowerment: A systematic review of measures. *PLoS ONE*, 10(5), pp.1–24.

Bergman-Chalmers, B. (2014). *Empathie empowering patients in the management of chronic diseases final summary report contract number*. 2013 62 01.

Bonsignore, C., Brolis, E., Ionescu, A., Karusinova, V., Mitkova, Z., Raps, F., Renman, V., & Ricci Fedotova, N. (2017). *Patient empowerment and centredness*. European Health Parliament. Available at: https://www.healthparliament.eu/wp-content/uploads/2017/09/EHP-papers_Patients-empowerment.pdf

Booth, R. G. (2006). Educating the future eHealth professional nurse. *International Journal of Nursing Education Scholarship*, 3(1), pp.1–10. Available at: http://www.degruyter.com/view/j/ijnes.2006.3.1/ijnes.2006.3.1.1187/ijnes.2006.3.1.1187.xml

Booth, R. G. (2016). Informatics and nursing in a post-nursing informatics world: Future directions for nurses in an automated, artificially intelligent, social-networked healthcare environment. *Canadian Journal of Nursing Leadership*, 28(4), pp.61–69.

Cerezo, P. G., Juvé-Udina, M. E. & Delgado-Hito, P. (2016). Concepts and measures of patient empowerment: A comprehensive review. *Revista da Escola de Enfermagem*, 50(4), pp.664–671.

Chen, Y.-C., & Li, I.-C. (2009). Effectiveness of interventions using empowerment concept for patients with chronic disease: A systematic review. *JBI Database of Systematic Reviews and Implementation Reports*, 7(27), pp.1179–1233.

Clancy, T. R. (2020). Artificial intelligence and nursing: The future is now. *The Journal of Nursing Administration*, 50(3), pp.125–127.

Coenen, A. (2003). The international classification for nursing practice (ICNP®) programme: Advancing a unifying framework for nursing. *The Online Journal of Issues in Nursing*, 8(2).

Crawford, A., & Serhal, E. (2020). Digital health equity and COVID-19: The innovation curve cannot reinforce the social gradient of health. *Journal of Medical Internet Research*, 22(6), pp.1–5.

Davenport, T., & Kalakota, R. (2019). The potential for artificial intelligence in healthcare. *Future Healthcare Journal*, 6(2), pp.94–98.

Dowding, D. W., Turley, M., & Garrido, T. (2014). Nurses' use of an integrated electronic health record: Results of a case site analysis. *Informatics for Health and Social Care*, 40(4), pp.345–361.

Eisenhauer, L. A., Hurley, A. C., & Dolan, N. (2007). Nurses' reported thinking during medication administration: Health policy and systems. *Journal of Nursing Scholarship*, 39(1), pp.82–87.

Garvin, J., Martin, K., Stassen, D., & Bowles, K. (2008). Omaha system: Coded data that describe patient care. *Journal of AHIMA*, 79(3), pp.44–49.

Health Promotion Glossary. (1998). Geneva: World Health Organization. Available at: https://www.who.int/healthpromotion/about/HPR%20Glossary%201998.pdf

Hulsen, T., Jamuar, S. S., Moody, A. R., Karnes, J. H., Varga, O., Hedensted, S., Spreafico, R., Hafler, D. A., & McKinney, E. F. (2019). From big data to precision medicine. *Frontiers in Medicine*, 6(Mar), p.34.

ICN and SNOMED sign ground-breaking agreement to secure a bright future for the International Classification for Nursing Practice. (2021). *SNOMED International*. Available at: https://www.snomed.org/news-and-events/articles/ICN-SNOMED-sign-groundbreaking-agreement-2020

Jerofke, T., Weiss, M., & Yakusheva, O. (2014). Patient perceptions of patient-empowering nurse behaviours, patient activation and functional health status in postsurgical patients with life-threatening long-term illnesses. *Journal of Advanced Nursing*, 70(6), pp.1310–1322.

Jones, D., Lunney, M., Keenan, G., & Moorhead, S. (2010). Standardized nursing languages essential for the nursing workforce. *Annual Review of Nursing Research*, 28, pp.253–294. https://doi.org/10.1891/0739-6686.28.253

Kambhampati, S., Ashvetiya, T., Stone, N. J., Blumenthal, R. S., & Martin, S. S. (2016). Shared decision-making and patient empowerment in preventive cardiology. *Current Cardiology Reports*, 18(5), pp.49–49.

Kemp, J., Zhang, T., Inglis, F., Wiljer, D., Sockalingam, S., Takhar, S. S., & Strudwick, G. (2020). Delivery of compassionate mental health care in a digital technology: Driven age: Scoping review. *Journal of Medical Internet Research*, 22(3), pp.1–15.

Keogh, J. (1997). Professionalization of nursing: Development, difficulties and solutions. *Journal of Advanced Nursing*, 25(2), pp.302–308.

Koekenbier, K., Leino-Kilpi, H., Cabrera, E., Istomina, N., Stark, Å. J., Katajisto, J., Lemonidou, C., Papastavrou, E., Salanterä, S., Sigurdardottir, A., Valkeapää, K., & Eloranta, S. (2016). Empowering knowledge and its connection to health-related quality of life: A cross-cultural study. A concise and informative title: Empowering knowledge and its connection to health-related quality of life. *Applied Nursing Research*, 29, pp.211–216.

Kossman, S. P., Bonney, L. A., & Kim, M. J. (2013). Electronic health record tools' support of nurses' clinical judgment and team communication. *CIN: Computers Informatics Nursing*, 31(11), pp.539–544.

Kostkova, P., Brewer, H., de Lusignan, S., Fottrell, E., Goldacre, B., Hart, G., Koczan, P., Knight, P., Marsolier, C., McKendry, R. A., Ross, E., Sasse, A., Sullivan, R., Chaytor, S., Stevenson, O., Velho, R., & Tooke, J. (2016). Who owns the data? Open data for healthcare. *Frontiers in Public Health*, 4. https://doi.org/10.3389/fpubh.2016.00007

Londoño, A. M. M., & Schulz, P. J. (2015). Influences of health literacy, judgment skills, and empowerment on asthma self-management practices. *Patient Education and Counseling*, 98(7), pp.908–917.

Matinolli, H. M., Mieronkoski, R., & Salanterä, S. (2020). Health and medical device development for fundamental care: Scoping review. *Journal of Clinical Nursing*, 29(11–12), pp.1822–1831.

McGrow, K. (2019). Artificial intelligence: Essentials for nursing. *Nursing*, 49(9), pp.46–49.

Meditskos, G., Vrochidis, S., & Kompatsiaris, I. (2017). Description logics and rules for multimodal situational awareness in healthcare. In *Lecture notes in computer science (including subseries lecture notes in artificial intelligence and lecture notes in bioinformatics)*. New York: Springer Verlag, pp.714–725.

Moen, H., Hakala, K., Peltonen, L.-M., Matinolli, H.-M., Suhonen, H., Terho, K., Danielsson-Ojala, R., Valta, M., Ginter, F., Salakoski, T., & Salanterä, S. (2020). Assisting nurses in care documentation: From automated sentence classification to coherent document structures with subject headings. *Journal of Biomedical Semantics* 11, p.10. https://doi.org/10.1186/s13326-020-00229-7

Morley, J., & Floridi, L. (2020). The limits of empowerment: How to reframe the role of mHealth tools in the healthcare ecosystem. *Science and Engineering Ethics*, 26(3), pp.1159–1183.

Motamedi, S. M., Posadas-Calleja, J., Straus, S., Bates, D. W., Lorenzetti, D. L., Baylis, B., Gilmour, J., Kimpton, S., & Ghali, W. A. (2011). The efficacy of computer-enabled discharge communication interventions: A systematic review. *BMJ Quality and Safety*, 20(5), pp.403–415.

Obermeyer, Z., Powers, B., Vogeli, C., & Mullainathan, S. (2019). Dissecting racial bias in an algorithm used to manage the health of populations. *Science*, 366(6464), pp.447–453.

Olson, P. (2014). *The quantified other: Nest and fitbit chase a lucrative side business*. Forbes. Available at: https://www.forbes.com/sites/parmyolson/2014/04/17/the-quantified-other-nest-and-fitbit-chase-a-lucrative-side-business/?sh=7d0700f82c8a

Pekonen, A., Eloranta, S., Stolt, M., Virolainen, P., & Leino-Kilpi, H. (2020). Measuring patient empowerment: A systematic review. *Patient Education and Counseling*, 103(4), pp.777–787.

Pepito, J. A., & Locsin, R. (2019). Can nurses remain relevant in a technologically advanced future? *International Journal of Nursing Sciences*, 6(1), pp.106–110.

Risling, T. (2017). Educating the nurses of 2025: Technology trends of the next decade. *Nurse Education in Practice*, 22, pp.89–92. https://doi.org/10.1016/j.nepr.2016.12.007

Risling, T., Martinez, J., Young, J., & Thorp-Froslie, N. (2017). Evaluating patient empowerment in association with eHealth technology: Scoping review. *Journal of Medical Internet Research*, 19, p.e329. https://doi.org/10.2196/jmir.7809

Rodriguez, J. A., Clark, C. R., & Bates, D. W. (2020). Digital health equity as a necessity in the 21st century cures act era. *JAMA: Journal of the American Medical Association*, 323(23), pp.2381–2382.

Rogers, M. L., Sockolow, P. S., Bowles, K. H., Hand, K. E., & George, J. (2013). Use of a human factors approach to uncover informatics needs of nurses in documentation of care. *International Journal of Medical Informatics*, 82, pp.1068–1074. https://doi.org/10.1016/j.ijmedinf.2013.08.007.

Ronquillo, C. E. et al. (May 2021). Artificial intelligence in nursing: Priorities and opportunities from an international invitational think-tank of the nursing and artificial intelligence leadership collaborative. *Journal of Advanced Nursing*, jan., p.14855.

Rutherford, M. (2008). Standardized nursing language: What does it mean for nursing practice? *The Online Journal of Issues in Nursing*, 13(1). Available at: https://ojin.nursingworld.org/MainMenuCategories/ThePracticeofProfessionalNursing/Health-IT/StandardizedNursingLanguage.html

Saranto, K., Kinnunen, U. M., Kivekäs, E., Lappalainen, A. M., Liljamo, P., Rajalahti, E., & Hyppönen, H. (2014). Impacts of structuring nursing records: A systematic review. *Scandinavian Journal of Caring Sciences*, 28(4), pp.629–647.

Shortliffe, E. H., & Sepúlveda, M. J. (2018). Clinical decision support in the era of artificial intelligence. *JAMA: Journal of the American Medical Association*, 320(21), pp.2199–2200.

Silberg, J., & Manyika, J. (2019). *Notes from the AI frontier: Tackling bias in AI (and in humans)*. McKinsey& Company. Available at: https://www.mckinsey.com/featured-insights/artificial-intelligence/tackling-bias-in-artificial-intelligence-and-in-humans

Sinha, C., & Schryer-Roy, A. M. (2018). Digital health, gender and health equity: Invisible imperatives. *Journal of Public Health*, 40(suppl_2), pp.II1–II5.

SNOMED CT. (2020). *SNOMED International*. https://www.snomed.org/snomed-ct/why-snomed-ct

Staggers, N., Gassert, C., & Curran, C. (2001). Informatics competencies for nurses at four levels of practice. *Journal of Nursing Education*, 40(7), pp.303–316.

Starmer, A. J., Sectish, T. C., Simon, D. W., Keohane, C., McSweeney, M. E., Chung, E. Y., Yoon, C. S., Lipsitz, S. R., Wassner, A. J., Harper, M. B., & Landrigan, C. P. (2013). Rates of medical errors and preventable adverse events among hospitalized children following implementation of a resident handoff bundle. *JAMA: Journal of the American Medical Association*, 310(21), pp.2262–2270.

Strudwick, G., Nagle, L., Kassam, I., Pahwa, M., & Sequeira, L. (2019). Informatics competencies for nurse leaders: A scoping review. *Journal of Nursing Administration*, 49(6), pp.323–330.

Topaz, M., Murga, L., Gaddis, K. M., McDonald, M. V., Bar-Bachar, O., Goldberg, Y., & Bowles, K. H. (2019). Mining fall-related information in clinical notes: Comparison of rule-based and novel word embedding-based machine learning approaches. *Journal of Biomedical Informatics*, 90, p.103103. https://doi.org/10.1016/j.jbi.2019.103103

Turing, A. M. (1950). Computing machinery and intelligence. *Mind*, LIX(236), pp.433–460.

Urquhart, C., & Currell, R. (2005). Reviewing the evidence on nursing record systems. *Health Informatics Journal*, 11(1), pp.33–44.

Urquhart, C., Currell, R., Grant, M. J., & Hardiker, N. R. (2009). Nursing record systems: Effects on nursing practice and healthcare outcomes. *Cochrane Database of Systematic Reviews*. https://doi.org/10.1002/14651858.CD002099.pub2

Were, M. C., Sinha, C., & Catalani, C. (2019). A systematic approach to equity assessment for digital health interventions: Case example of mobile personal health records. *Journal of the American Medical Informatics Association*, 26, pp.884–890. https://doi.org/10.1093/jamia/ocz071

Wiljer, D., Charow, R., Costin, H., Sequeira, L., Anderson, M., Strudwick, G., Tripp, T., & Crawford, A. (2019). Defining compassion in the digital health age: Protocol for a scoping review. *BMJ Open*, 9(2), pp.1–7.

World Health Organization. (n.d.). *WHO releases new international classification of diseases (ICD 11)*. Available at: https://www.who.int/news/item/18-06-2018-who-releases-new-international-classification-of-diseases-(icd-11)

World Health Organization & Office for Europe Region. (2013). *Health 2020: A European policy framework supporting action across government and society for health and well-being.*

Yu, P., Zhang, Y., Gong, Y., & Zhang, J. (2013). Unintended adverse consequences of introducing electronic health records in residential aged care homes. *International Journal of Medical Informatics*, 82(9), pp.772–788.

Ziebarth, D. J. (2018). Exploring standardized nursing languages: Moving toward a faith community nursing intervention. *International Journal of Faith Community Nursing*, 4(1).

Chapter 4

Ethical Considerations in Digital Health

Pirkko Kouri, Minna Kaija-Kortelainen,
Margaret Ann Kennedy and Riitta Turjamaa

Contents

Introduction

Ethics can be defined as the starting point for respecting and protecting life-reasoning skills and as guidelines for assessing the realization of public and private good in an inviolable manner. At its simplest, ethics deals with good and evil, values and norms, rights and responsibilities. The domain of ethics has a strong liaison with morality (FNA, 2021; Ellemers et al., 2019; Drobnickij, 1975). The concept of ethics and the content of ethics are broader than morality because it includes moral reflection and morality research (FNA, 2021; Stokhof, 2018; ETENE, 2002). Ethics and morals refer

DOI: 10.4324/9781003054849-4

to habits, customs and limitations that regulate people's mutual lives (FNA, 2021; West, 2019; Shahriari et al., 2013, ETENE, 2009). Based on their literature review, Shahriari et al. (2013) suggest the following nursing ethical values, which are human dignity, justice, privacy, autonomy in decision making, precision and accuracy in caring, commitment, human relationship, honesty and individual and professional competency, for instance. Ethics describes and justifies good and right ways of living and working in the world, which man shares with others (Singer, 2021; ETENE, 2002). Furthermore, universal and widespread ethics principles adopted are non-harm, benefit generation, fairness and equality, dignity and feasibility (Singer, 2021; FNA, 2021; Henk et al., 2009). When values and norms conflict with each other, an ethical problem arises.

Foundations of Ethics in a Digital World

Recently, Malkavaara (2020) stated that there are four starting points for morality and ethics. Firstly, life is the most important good; it is valued and it is defended. Secondly, morality concerns human nature and human deeds. Thirdly, a person works for their own benefit and to realize their own good by nature. Lastly, morality is about a person's relationship with other people and the environment. Ethical rules and orders are not just external laws, but based on conscience, the integrity of internal information, to the innermost sanctuary of conscience, to a quiet conscience call or firm faith (FNA, 2021; WHO, 2017; ETENE, 2002). Addressing the ethical issues brought by digitalization requires different perspectives and multidisciplinary discussions between experts (FNA, 2021; ANA, 2018).

According to Royakkers et al. (2018), visible and invisible technology is around us in every aspect of our lives: the technology embedded itself in us (e.g., through brain implants), between us through social media (e.g., Twitter, Facebook), learns and thus knows more and more about us via AI, big data and techniques such as emotion recognition and is constantly learning and adopting our behavior like human or animal-like robots that can mimic emotions and be connected by producing voice (Royakkers et al., 2018; Niculescu et al., 2013). Increasingly, organizations are using fingerprint and facial recognition to make their services more convenient and to improve security. This leads to the fact that citizens are waking up to the fact that their information is being collected by both different entities and have begun to demand control and transparency (Malkavaara, 2020; Nabbosa & Kaar, 2020; Love, 2011). Technology is not just a supporter of healthcare; it shapes the field of healthcare. It is important to broaden the perspective on, for example, how virtual and augmented reality or the internet of things live in the future. Furthermore, data-intensive software, such as social media solutions, wellness and mobile health apps, have become ubiquitous in everyday life and are frequently used in a variety of situations. The possibility of invisible health data complicates the situation further. It is challenging how citizens and patients in the social and health sectors capable of functioning in different operating environments take over equally new remote-control tools. There is a need for universal data protection and comprehensive consent (Malkavaara, 2020; Schneble et al., 2020; Nabbosa & Kaar, 2020; WHO, 2017).

Today, more and more hacking, cyber-attacks and other forms of cyber-crime are on the rise, creating real threats to organizations. Simultaneously with necessary digitalization, criminals are developing their own activities faster and more efficiently, so new secured means of protection must be found (Jang & Nepal, 2014). Exponential growth in the types of versatile data that are collected and their interlinkages are enabling more predictions of individuals' health status, behavior and diseases. Organizations should take care of a range of issues such as risk management, security and information policy, security of human resources, qualified access control, and information security incidence management (Schneble et al., 2020; Yang, 2018). It is important to have a constant ethical reflection on the evaluation of right and wrong environments of virtual data management.

Social media is challenging nurses. Nurses write blogs and tweets, participate in virtual networking sites and use online chats and forums to express themselves both personally and professionally with others. Social media is a valuable tool when used wisely. The use of social media has included an unwritten law that nurses should distinguish between different aspects of social media: does she/he act as an individual on social media or as a nurse representing an employer or profession. In addition, the unsuitable use of social media by nurses may result in revealing too much information and violate patient privacy and confidentiality. Nurses should carefully consider whether joining a patient or client network is even possible as an individual (NCSBN, 2018; cf. Act on the Status and Rights of Patients, 1992).

Based on the Act on the Status and Rights of Patients (1992), every nurse who deals with a patient's healthcare data must have legal access and the right to process patient data. When nurses are accessing patient data, they must ensure that they are following acceptable user policy as stated by the healthcare organization and not leave data (for example, files) open when not taking care of the patient. In addition, the nurse who has no working relationship with a patient is considered as an outsider who is not allowed to use secured patient information (Love, 2011). Technological development and communication-related information are quickly and efficiently transferable, storable and reusable. The use of digital technology presents numerous opportunities for improving and transforming healthcare which include minimizing human errors, improving care outcomes, facilitating healthcare coordination, improving practice efficiencies and tracking data over time (EU, 2020; Alotaibi & Federico, 2017).

Most people are just users in relation to digital solutions and artificial intelligence (AI). It has been anticipated that networked AI will amplify human effectiveness but also threaten human autonomy, agency and capabilities (EU, 2020; Anderson & Rainie, 2018). The rapid development of learning machines or artificial intelligence has since heightened fear that a new generation of machines is emerging that is able to think and can therefore supplant humans (Dufva, 2020). Robotics refers to many types of devices that can be programmed to perform desired sequences of motion, often in relation to the device's observations of the environment. Instead of AI, we could talk about programs that take advantage of machine learning. AI applications replace and complement human activity even more radically because they are programmed to learn and develop themselves. They can be used to collect the most diverse data, aggregate, compare and evaluate as programs develop new ways to improve their own operations. It is no longer just a matter of speed and scope of huge data processing, but AI makes digital systems creative (Thomas, 2020; EU, 2020; Anderson & Rainie, 2018; Niculescu et al., 2013).

Constant monitoring challenges every person's privacy issues. From the viewpoint of patients, related to one's health information, there are 'four Ws': *who* wants to know *what, from whom* and for *what reason*. A person should be able to monitor their health data processing in real-time and stay informed on the phase and scope of the processing of their data; be given an opportunity to withdraw their consent in real-time; have a guarantee that data is protected by default; have the authority to control who, why and for what purpose their data is used (Hämäläinen et al., 2020).

Case Study Finland: Novel Ethical Operation's Model Developed in a National Project

In Finland, there was a national project called SOTEPEDA 24/7, during 2018–2020, which was funded by the Finnish Ministry of Education and Culture. The ethical model is a qualitative description of the way in how work can be delineated or a nursing task performed. The model defines the idea, purpose, target group, description and concrete use of the operational model and its benefits. One of the project's goals was to create an ethical action model for digital services in the health and social care sector.

The model concretely illustrates the elements and knowledge that are strongly linked with ethical activities and problem-solving in an increasingly digitized operational, social and healthcare domain. Anticipating future changes prepares staff for new ethical challenges. The ethical model consists of five sections (see Figure 4.1) that form a holistic ground, in which the areas are interactive with each other. The process of the ethical model can be utilized at the level of the individual/employee, work community, organization and society (Sihvo et al., 2021).

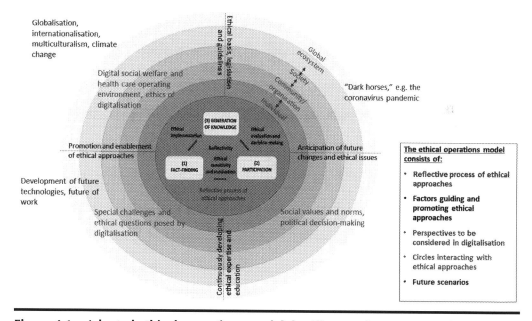

Figure 4.1   Adapted ethical operations model, by Sihvo et al. 2021, p. 9 (Licensed by CC BY-NC-SA).

CASE STUDY CANADA: SOCIAL MEDIA USE BY NURSES

Social media has been an invaluable tool to many innovative healthcare initiatives; however, a lack of guidance on the appropriate use of social media has led to conflicts between provincial nursing regulators and individual clinicians. Such is the case of nurse Carolyn Strom from Saskatchewan, Canada, who posted a lengthy comment on Facebook in 2015 about the quality of care her late grandfather received during the last weeks and months of his life. She was off duty when she posted a comment as a family member of the deceased about how the staff at St. Joseph's integrated Health Centre needed to improve the care of their elderly patients.

The provincial nursing regulator, the Saskatchewan Registered Nurses Association, alleged that by calling out the named organization and staff, Ms. Strom had committed a violation of professional standards of practice. In 2016, the Association found her guilty of professional misconduct and ordered her to pay a $1,000 fine and $25,000 in tribunal fees (Sciarpelletti, 2020). Following this decision, civil liberty groups, individual nurses and the Saskatchewan Nurses Union all contacted her to offer support. Confusion was high during this time, but there was outrage over the infringement of individual rights to post on social media outside of one's professional role.

Ms. Strom appealed the regulator's guilty verdict and fine to the Court of Queen's Bench; however, this appeal was dismissed in 2018. She then appealed to the Saskatchewan Court of Appeals. This Court ruled that her rights to free speech were unjustifiably infringed and that she had a right to criticize her grandfather's care (Sciarpelletti, 2020). The Appeals judge also noted that criticism of the healthcare systems is in the public interest, and that criticism from front-line staff can often bring positive results.

This case study, while demonstrating the priority of free speech, also illustrates the gap in clear guidance on the use of social media by clinicians, which has the potential to result in ethical violations. While posting photos of patients or divulging patient-related data are clear violations of privacy as governed by privacy laws in Canada (Government of Canada, 2019a, b) and the Canadian Nurses Association Code of Ethics (2008), these are types of gross privacy violations that have occurred early on in the advent of social media and have diminished over time.

Past presentations at the national level hosted by the Canadian Nurses Association (Newton & Guitard, 2009) focused on the ethical use of social media from a fundamental perspective of privacy, appropriate use during work hours and access to social media as a social justice issue but did little to elevate the larger conversation about the ethical use of social media or address some of the nuances of social media use.

There is no single definitive national position statement on ethics and social media in Canada, and although the Canadian Nurses Association Code of Ethics addresses technology broadly, it does not mention social media explicitly. Instead, provincial regulators of nursing (for example, Nova Scotia College of Nurses, n.d.; College of Registered Nurses of Newfoundland, 2013) have developed practice guidelines and learning modules that help to prepare nurses about expectations of professional use and social media, although this type of guidance is not available in all provinces across Canada. The International Nurse Regulator Collaborative (INRC, 2016) also released a set of common expectations of nurses when using social media, but it is unclear if this is promoted and enforced robustly in all member bodies. Along with Nursing Boards from Australia, New Zealand, Ireland, Singapore and the USA, only two of Canada's 13 regulatory colleges for registered nurses hold membership in the INRC, illustrating the persistent gap in guidance and exposing a risk of future ethical conflicts.

Safe Digital Health and Older People

The majority of older people are healthy and are living independently in their own homes for longer (de Bruin et al., 2018). Therefore, there is a growing interest in using digital solutions to support older people's living at home, assist them in everyday activities and improve their quality of life (Sharkey & Sharkey, 2012).

Digital solutions for older people include different kinds of communication and network systems, such as applications, sensors and monitors (Cook, 2012). In addition, digital solutions have experience when collecting data on older people's physical activity at home, such as making coffee and realizing everyday activities, such as using lights, doors and windows (Austin et al., 2016). In addition, social robots have been used to improve social contact and to decrease loneliness and as domestic aids to assess daily activities, such as taking care of medication, eating, bathing and getting dressed (Wu et al., 2014).

In recent years, there is a growing interest in using robots to help older people with everyday activities. However, significant ethical questions are important to consider when supporting older people's living at home using robotics and also other smart home technology (Draper & Sorell, 2017, Sánchez et al., 2017). Data security and views of privacy use of digital solutions in older people's home care raise questions about which data are collected at home, for example, by using sensors and cameras, and how data is kept, who owns it and what happens to that (Sánchez et al., 2017). If digital solutions are not able to discern the difference between confidential information (e.g., personal health information) and information that the user permits for release, then the robot may violate a user's privacy.

Privacy can be described in several perspectives and dimensions, such as informational, social and physical privacy (Stahl & Coeckelbergh, 2016). From the perspective of autonomy, using digital solutions enabling older people to perform their everyday activities independently are important elements to supporting and maintaining autonomy (Stahl & Coeckelbergh, 2016). Autonomy also emphasizes the right to make decisions based on the use of digital solutions as a part their daily care (Jacobs, 2018). However, older people may not be capable of making decisions about the abilities and limitations of an offered digital solutions about the abilities and limitations of a robot technology and be aware of his or her own possibly biased perceptions of it (Draper & Sorell, 2017). The loss of autonomy can also influence older people's sense of personal dignity (Sharkey, 2014).

Digital solutions for older people's safety are related to physical circumstances at home, physical activity and social isolation and loneliness. These points are especially important in-home care, since it often involves vulnerable people with physical and cognitive disabilities (Brims & Oliver, 2018). Therefore, it is essential to take into account older people's rights to self-determination in the context of making decisions about their care and use of digital solutions at home.

A lot of different data is emerging today about health. People both produce it actively, but data is generated passively also. Passive data arises when different devices, for example, are collecting and storing it, without the user itself actively producing it (Maher et al., 2019, p. 242). There should be ethical and legal guidelines for sharing data (Hollis, 2016).

Different health-related applications have been developed for smartphones, which play a significant role in communicating with patients through various applications (Mosa et al., 2012). New forms of personal health data (PHD) collection are creating new requirements for privacy. Information is more easily shared in different social media channels, for example (Bietz et al., 2016, p. 42). Citizens use health technology to measure things related to health or activity. However, this exploitation of measured information raises questions. The majority of the public would like to self-manage the health data (or MyData) they collect (MyData in Healthcare –survey, 2019). Current practices and legislation have been created for examining official health information produced and stored in official health archives (Bietz et al., 2016, 47).

According to research, people are willing to share information (data) anonymously for the common good (Bietz et al., 2016, 45, 47). The data will revolutionize research and treatment practices because it is now easy for patients and customers to gather a lot of information for treatment and research (Carter et al., 2015). The most vulnerable clients or patients will not be able to benefit from this tracking of their own data because they do not have access to mHealth technology or other technology (Carter et al., 2015). In particular, there are challenges to inactive data in terms of people not understanding the consent they make, for example, when downloading a health file to their phone for example (Balestra et al., 2016). However, information collected on the phone about one's health or well-being may not be secret; it could be accessed by hackers or authorities (Carter et al., 2015).

Ownership and the Patient's Role in Producing Social and Healthcare Data

Who actually owns the data written by a professional about the patient stored in a state-owned or hospital-owned database? Informational privacy includes the right to prescribe information concerning oneself (Saarenpää, 2007). The patient, therefore, has the primary right to prescribe information concerning themselves, to keep secret information about himself, the right to share information about himself, the right to influence the use of information and the right to inspect the data. In addition to this, the person has the right to disclose information about himself, influence the release of his own information and the right to correct errors in the information (Voutilainen, 2019, Leino-Kilpi et al., 2001).

However, there has been little discussion to date about the role of the patient as an active producer of information. What kind of risk (e.g., security) is involved when a patient shares their own data and documentation via their own phone? Is the data generated by the patient correct? How and for what purposes do professionals use the patient's own produced information?

CASE STUDY—KANTA DIGITAL ARCHIVING SERVICES FOR THE SOCIAL WELFARE AND HEALTHCARE SECTOR

Social and healthcare data, medical records and prescriptions are recorded in Kanta. Today, a patient can give consent to the release of their medical records to other healthcare units, and if they wish, to limit the scope of consent with prohibitions. Medical records stored in Kanta are available to the healthcare unit that entered the information. The patient's consent is required when data is used in another unit. The My Kanta portal also enables, for example, to monitor your own health data, prescriptions and well-being data. The My Kanta portal allows you to store information about various wellness applications and devices into My Kanta (Kanta, 2021).

The extensive electronic use of the client data allows for a smooth customer process. However, the wide use of information also allows for misuse. In electronic information systems, it is also possible to limit on the basis of work tasks who has the right to look at and what client data is accessible. This, however, does not fully eliminate the possibility of malpractice. What is problematic from a client's fundamental rights and privacy point of view is that monitoring of the use of client data is ex post facto. However, no technical system will be able to guarantee that data will not be misused, but ultimately the question is the ethics of professionals. Electronic archives and technology bring not only security but also new risks.

Many countries are interested in using electronic health and social records. The big question is: how we can utilize technological advances and at the same time find a balance between the many competing interests around health and personal privacy (Presser et al., 2015). However, in many countries, there is no separate legislation, but privacy law defines how data can be used (Deloitte, 2016, p. 48). The secondary use of social and health data relates to information collected for primary use but is being utilized for other purposes. The primary use of personal data refers to the purpose for which the data was initially stored when providing healthcare or social welfare services (Deloitte, 2016, 3,4). The secondary data can be utilized for service planning, guidance, monitoring and research.

The risks associated with the secondary use of social and healthcare data have not been adequately aware. Furthermore, the implications of data and its use have not been discussed, taking into account the wider also controversial social impacts. Many data harms have been noticed, for example, privacy breaches, discrimination and stigma, disenfranchisement, disempowerment and exploitation (Ballantyne, 2020). Data usage should have the original purpose for which it was collected. Authoritarian governments can also misuse data. The technology will be able to protect data. However, it is not possible to protect data if politicians change legislation to change the use of the data (O'Doherty, 2016). Transparency is the most important thing when utilizing data for secondary purposes.

Conclusion

Digital health is integrated into a complex network of different parties, involving not only the users and providers of digital health technologies and applications. Today, the role of patients is changing due to the growing participation of healthcare via digital tools. There are challenges regarding safe access in digital health services, truthful information sharing to end-users, dignity and fairness in storage, data sharing and ownership of data, and demand of fully informed consent. Digital health providers and regulators should ensure that digital health interventions are designed and set up in an ethical and fair way and foster health equity for all user groups. In addition, nurses should have skills to assess the benefits, harms, acceptability, resource use and equity considerations of digital health interventions.

References

Act on the Status and Rights of Patients. (785/1992). Available at: https://finlex.fi/en/laki/kaannokset/1992/en19920785

Alotaibi, Y. K., & Federico, F. (2017 December). The impact of health information technology on patient safety. *Saudi Medical Journal*, 38(12), pp.1173–1180. https://doi.org/10.15537/smj.2017.12.20631. PMID: 29209664; PMCID: PMC5787626. Available at: https://smj.org.sa/content/38/12/1173

Anderson, J., & Rainie, L. (2018). *Artificial intelligence and the future of humans.* Pew Research Center. Internet & Technology. Available at: https://www.pewresearch.org/internet/2018/12/10/artificial-intelligence-and-the-future-of-humans/

Austin, J., Dodge, H. H., Riley, T., Jacobs, P. G., Thielke, S., & Kaye, J. (2016). A smart-home system to unobtrusively and continuously assess loneliness in older adults. *IEEE Journal of Translational Engineering in Health and Medicine*, 4, pp.1–8. [online]. Available at: https://doi.org/10.1109/JTEHM.2016.2579638.

Balestra, M., Shaer, O., Okerlund, J., Westendorf, L., Ball, M., & Nov, O. (2016). Social annotation valence: The impact on online informed consent beliefs and behavior. *Journal of Medical Internet Research*, 18, p.e197. https://doi.org/10.2196/jmir.5662

Ballantyne, A. (2020). How should we think about clinical data ownership? *Journal of Medical Ethics*, 46, pp.289–294.

Bietz, M. J., Bloss, C. S., Calvert, S., Godino, J. G., Gregory, J., Claffey, M. P., Sheehan, J., & Patrick, K. (2016). Opportunities and challenges in the use of personal health data for health research. *Journal of the American Medical Informatics Association*, 23, pp.e42–e48. https://doi.org/10.1093/jamia/ocv118

Brims, L., & Oliver, K. (2018). Effectiveness of assistive technology in improving the safety of people with dementia: A systematic review and meta-analysis. *Aging & Mental Health*, 23(8), pp.942–951.

Canadian Nurses Association. (2008). Code of ethics for registered nurses. https://www.cna-aiic.ca/-/media/cna/page-content/pdf-en/code_of_ethics_2008_e.pdf

Carter, A., Liddle, J., Hall, W., & Chenery, H. (2015). Mobile phones in research and treatment: Ethical guidelines and future directions. *JMIR mHealth uHealth*, 3(4), p.e95 doi: 10.2196/mhealth.4538

College of Registered Nurses of Newfoundland. (2013). *Social media*. Available at: https://www.crnnl.ca/sites/default/files/documents/ID_Social_Media.pdf

Cook, D. J. (2012). How smart is your home? *Science*, 335(6076), pp.1579–1581.

de Bruin, S. R., Stoop, A., Billings, J., Leichsenring, K., Ruppe, G., Tram, N., & Baan, C. A. (2018). The SUSTAIN project: A European study on improving integrated care for older people living at home. *International Journal of Integrated Care*, 18(1), pp.1–12.

Deloitte: Holland, C. (n.d.). *International privacy day global privacy - 2016, the Year of Reform 6*. Available at: https://www2.deloitte.com/content/dam/Deloitte/za/Documents/legal/za_Legal-Update-Issue-1.pdf

Draper, H., & Sorell, T. (2017). Ethical values and social care robots for older people: An international qualitative study. *Ethics and Information Technology*, 19(1), pp.49–68.

Drobnickij, O. (1975). Ethics. In T. J. Blakeley, eds., *Themes in soviet marxist philosophy. Sovietica (publications and monographs of the institute of East-European Studies at the University of Fribourg/Switzerland and the Center for East Europe, Russia and Asia at Boston College and the Seminar for Political Theory and Philosophy at the University of Munich)*, vol 37. Dordrecht: Springer. https://doi.org/10.1007/978-94-010-1873-9_10

Dufva, M. (2020). *The big picture of the megatrends. Foresight. Sitra*. Available at: https://www.sitra.fi/en/articles/the-big-picture-of-the-megatrends

Ellemers, N., van der Toorn, J., Paunov, Y., & van Leeuwen, T. (2019, Sep/Oct). The psychology of morality: A review and analysis of empirical studies published from 1940 through 2017. *Personality and Social Psychology Review,* 23(4), pp.332–366. https://doi.org/10.1177/1088868318811759. Epub 2019 Jan 18. PMID: 30658545; PMCID: PMC6791030.

ETENE (The National Advisory Board on Social Welfare and Health Care Ethics). (2002). *The Parliamentary Ombudsmen's request for opinion. Statements and opinions.* Available at: https://etene.fi/en/statements-and-opinions-2002

ETENE (The National Advisory Board on Social Welfare and Health Care Ethics). (2009). *Measures to protect and restrict a patient's right of self-determination. Statements and opinions.* Available at: https://etene.fi/en/statements-and-opinions-2009

European Union (EU). (2020, March). The ethics of artificial intelligence: Issues and initiatives. *Study panel for the future of science and technology.* European Parliamentary Research Service. Scientific Foresight Unit (STOA). PE 634.452. Available online at: https://www.europarl.europa.eu/RegData/etudes/STUD/2020/634452/EPRS_STU(2020)634452_EN.pdf

Finnish Nurse Association (FNA). (2021). *Code of ethics for nurses.* Updated Spring. Available at: https://sairaanhoitajat.fi/wp-content/uploads/2021/04/Code-of-Ethics-for-Nurses-2021.pdf

Government of Canada. (2019a). Privacy act. Bill C-21. Department of Justice. http://laws-lois.justice.gc.ca/eng/acts/P-21/

Government of Canada. (2019b). *Personal information protection and electronic documents Act.* Bill C-6. Department of Justice. Available at: http://laws-lois.justice.gc.ca/eng/acts/P-8.6/index.html

Hämäläinen, H., Malkamäki, S., Räsänen, I., Sinipuro, J., & Olesch, A. (2020). *Towards trustworthy health data ecosystems. How the reuse of data can create new services for the benefit of all.* Sitra working paper. Sitra. Available at: https://media.sitra.fi/2020/10/08101601/towards-trustworthy-health-data-ecosystems-2.pdf

ten Have, H. A. M. J., & Jean, M. S., eds. (2009). The UNESCO universal declaration on bioethics and human rights, background, principles and applications. *Ethics Series.* Published by the United Nations Educational, Scientific and Cultural Organization. Available at: http://www.unesco-chair-bioethics.org/wp-content/uploads/2015/08/The-UNESCO-Universal-Declaration-on-Bioethics-and-Human-Rights-Background-Principles-and-Application.pdf

Hollis, K. F. (2016). To share or not to share: Ethical acquisition and use of medical data. *AMIA Summits on Translational Science Proceedings,* 2016, pp.420–427. Google Scholar

International Nurse Regulator Collaborative (2016, December). *Social media use: Common expectations for nurses.* Available at: https://www.cno.org/globalassets/docs/prac/incr-social-media-use-common-expectations-for-nurses.pdf

Jacobs, G. (2018). Patient autonomy in home care: Nurses' relational practices of responsibility. *Nursing Ethics,* 26(6), pp.1638–1653.

Jang-Jaccard, J., & Nepal, S. (2014). A survey of emerging threats in cybersecurity. *Journal of Computer and System Sciences*, 80(5), pp.973–993. https://doi.org/10.1016/j.jcss.2014.02.005.

Kanta (2021). Available at: https://www.kanta.fi/en/citizens

Leino-Kilpi, H, Välimäki, M, Dassen, T, Gasull, M, Lemonidou, C, Scott, A, Arndt, M. (2001). Privacy: A review of the literature. *International Journal of Nursing Studies*, 38(6), pp.663–671. ISSN 0020-7489. https://doi.org/10.1016/S002 0-7489(00)00111-5.

Love, V. (2011). Privacy ethics in healthcare. *Journal of Healthcare Compliance.* Available at: https://www.researchgate.net/publication/283721153_Privacy _Ethics_in_Healthcare

Maher, N. A., Senders, J. T., Hulsbergen, A. F. C., Lamba, N., Parker, M., Onnela, J.-P., Bredenoord, A. L., Smith, T. R., & Broekman, M. L. D. (2019). Passive data collection and use in healthcare: A systematic review of ethical issues. *International Journal of Medical Informatics*, 129(September), pp.242–247.

Malkavaara, M. (n.d.). Johdatus etiikkaan (in English: Introduction to Ethics) in the book. In P. Sihvo, & A. Koski, eds., *Ethical operations model: Competence for future education and work in the field of social services and health care*, pp 52–60. Only abstract in English. Publications of Karelia University of Applied Sciences. B:65. ISBN 978-952-275-314-4 [online]. Available at: https://www.researchgate.net/profile/Paeivi-Sihvo/publication/349164073_Eettinen_toimin-tamalli/links/6023d44592851c4ed56160c2/Eettinen-toimintamalli.pdf (English translation of the book is coming soon).

Mosa, A. S. M., Yoo, I., & Sheets, L.. (2012). A systematic review of healthcare applications for smartphones. *BMC Medical Informatics Decision Making*, 12, p.67. https://doi.org/10.1186/1472-6947-12-67

MyData terveydenhuollossa –kyselytutkimus. (2019). *Kestävä Terveydenhuolto – hanke*. Sustainable Healthcare Project. Available at: https://www.tehy.fi/fi/system/files/mfiles/muu_dokumentti/mydata_raportti_web_id_14333.pdf (Accessed 1.6.2021).

Nabbosa, V., & Kaar, C. (2020). *Societal and ethical issues of digitalization*. https://doi.org/10.1145/3437075.3437093. Available at: https://www.researchgate.net/publication/346170706_Societal_and_Ethical_Issues_of_Digitalization

NCSBN. 2018. *A nurse's guide to the use of social media*. Available at: https://www.ncsbn.org/NCSBN_SocialMedia.pdf

Newton, L., & Guitard, V. (2009). Exploring the ethics of social media. CNA webinar series: Progress in practice. Available at: https://www.cna-aiic.ca/-/media/cna/page-content/pdf-en/social-media-webinar-march2012_e.pdf

Niculescu, A., van Dijk, B., & Nijholt, A. et al. Making social robots more attractive: The effects of voice pitch, humor and empathy. *International Journal of Social Robotics*, 5, pp.171–191 (2013).

Nova Scotia College of Nurses (n.d.). *Social media practice guideline*. Available at: https://cdn1.nscn.ca/sites/default/files/documents/resources/Social_Media .pdf

O'Doherty, K. C., Christofides, E., Yen, J., Bentzen, H. B., Burke, W., Hallowell, N., Koenig, B. A., & Willison, D. J. (2016). If you build it, they will come: Unintended future uses of organised health data collections. *BMC Medical Ethics*, 17, p.54. https://doi.org/10.1186/s12910-016-0137-x

Presser, L., Hruskova, M., Rowbottom, H., & Kancir, J. (2015). *Care data and access to UK health records: Patient privacy and public trust.* Available at: https://tech-science.org/a/2015081103/

Royakkers, L., Timmer, J., Kool, L., & van Est, R. (2018). Societal and ethical issues of digitization. *Ethics and Information Technology*, 20, pp.127–142. https://doi.org/10.1007/s10676-018-9452-x

Saarenpää, A. (2007). Informaatio-oikeus. s. 1–110 teoksessa Haavisto, Risto (toim.). Oikeusjärjestys. Osa 1. 5., täydennetty painos. Lapin yliopiston oikeustieteellisiä julkaisuja, sarja C 47. Lapin yliopisto.

Sánchez, V. G., Taylor, I., & Bing-Johnsson, P. C. (2017). Ethics of smart house welfare technology for older adults: A systematic literature review. *International Journal of Technology Assessment in Health Care*, 33(6), pp.691–699.

Schneble, C. O., Elger, B. S., & Shaw, D. M. (2020). All our data will be health data one day: The need for universal data protection and comprehensive consent. *Journal of Medical Internet Research*, 22(5), p.e16879. https://doi.org/10.2196/16879

Sciarpelletti, L. (2020, Oct 6). Sask nurse who was disciplined over Facebook comments wins court appeal. *CBC News*. Available at: https://www.cbc.ca/news/canada/saskatchewan/sask-nurse-carolyn-strom-wins-appeal-1.5752592

Shahriari, M., Mohammadi, E., Abbaszadeh, A., & Bahrami, M. (2013, Jan). Nursing ethical values and definitions: A literature review. *Iranian Journal of Nursing and Midwifery Research*, 18(1), pp.1–8. PMID: 23983720; PMCID: PMC3748548.

Sharkey, A. (2014). Robots and human dignity: A consideration of the effects of robot care on the dignity of older people. *Ethics and Information Technology*, 16(1), pp.63–75.

Sharkey, A., & Sharkey, N. (2012). Granny and the robots: Ethical issues in robot care for the elderly. *Ethics and Information Technology*, 14(1), pp.27–40.

Sihvo, P., Vesterinen, O., Koski, A., Malkavaara, M., & Pasanen, M. (2021). Ethical operational model at the core of competence. In *Handbooks and article collections: 70*. Joensuu: Publications of Karelia University of Applied Sciences B.

Singer, P. (2021). Ethics. *Encyclopedia Britannica*, 2 Feb. 2021. Available at: https://www.britannica.com/topic/ethics-philosophy (Accessed 23 April 2021).

Stahl, B. C., & Coeckelbergh, M. (2016). Ethics of healthcare robotics: Towards responsible research and innovation. *Robotics and Autonomous Systems*, 86, pp.152–161.

Stokhof, M. J. B. (2018). Ethics and morality, principles and practice. *ZEMO* 1, pp.291–304. https://doi.org/10.1007/s42048-018-0016-x

Thomas, M. (2020). *The future of robots and robotics*. Available at: https://builtin.com/robotics/future-robots-robotics

Voutilainen, T. (2019). Oikeus tietoon, Informaatio-oikeuden perusteet. (2. uudistettu painos).Edita.

West, E. (2019). Ethics and integrity in nursing research. In R. Iphofen, eds., *Handbook of research ethics and scientific integrity.* Cham: Springer. https://doi.org/10.1007/978-3-319-76040-7_46-

WHO. (2017). Code of ethics and professional conduct. Available at: https://www.who.int/about/ethics/code_of_ethics_full_version.pdf

Wu, Y.-H., Wrobel, J., Cornuet, M., Kerhervé, H., Damnée, S., & Rigaud, A.-S. (2014). Acceptance of an assistive robot in older adults: A mixed-method study of human–robot interaction over a 1-month period in the Living Lab setting. *Clinical Interventions in Aging*, 8(9), pp.801–811.

Yang, Y. (2018). *Literature review of information security practice survey reports.* Master's Thesis. Service Innovation and Management. University of Jyväskylä, 2018. Available at: https://jyx.jyu.fi/bitstream/handle/123456789/59443/URN:NBN:fi:jyu-201809064034.pdf;jsessionid=30F47666AFEC981931F22E07C965C4A9?sequence=1

Chapter 5

US Health and Healthcare Current State: Nurse Executives

Robyn Begley, Laura Reed and Julibeth Lauren

Contents

Introduction

What is digital transformation in healthcare? This question has been posed to many, especially in the last 18 months or more, and yet everyone defines transformation differently. Fueled by the pandemic over the last 18 months, we have experienced a change in our digital platform, which is unprecedented from the previous ten years of practice. Yet we know healthcare has still significantly lagged behind in implementing digital strategies as

DOI: 10.4324/9781003054849-5

compared to banking, airlines and other consumer-based buying (Jones et al., 2019).

Digital transformation for nursing, and healthcare in general, is an essential building block for patient-centered care. It helps to streamline day-to-day care and understand our patients' wishes or preferences in their plan of care. That deep connection builds loyalty and trust with our patients and community. It also improves the work life of our teams and clinicians, where they are asked to deliver care in very complex and challenging environments.

Digital transformation is now being demanded by our consumers. Most, if not all, consumers are open to and prefer digital offerings (Business Wire). This could include anything from searching for a physician or provider to payment functions, monitoring of daily health metrics, searching for costs or scheduling appointments.

The COVID-19 pandemic accelerated the shift in consumer demand and behavior to seek non-traditional care delivery models (Research & Markets, 2021). We quickly saw a dramatic change in the need for virtual emergency options and for convenience for on-demand care. Consumers of healthcare services needed to have convenient, connected and responsive services without actually physically visiting an office or clinic.

While the need for big data interactions to predict care and prevent human errors has been an expectation, we had failed to realize the degree to which we had/have opportunities for improvement. Consumers also want to be provided real-time alerts through wearable devices to prevent admissions/readmissions and to improve overall health and well-being (Takyar, n.d.). Big data provides this information to ensure the capacity to follow the best practice and implement targeted strategies for populations and strategic planning. During COVID-19, artificial intelligence was critical for understanding anticipated patient volumes, given the COVID-19 positivity rate and hospitalizations. COVID-19 also enabled adding multiple variables to the data captured and used, including personal protective equipment, ventilators, ICU and Medical Surgical bed capacity plus, most importantly, the number of staff needed or available. This real-time use of data technology and predictive analytics allowed health systems to respond to unprecedented events with as much knowledge as available.

The pandemic increased the needs for remote communications between patients and staff, patients and families and between systems. The adoption of telehealth, digital and mobile applications quickly drove adoption and adaptation to advance a consumer to business healthcare, thus moving from traditional healthcare systems mode of providing services and doing business.

The chronic disease needs are especially interesting as patients have had to improve their own health and well-being without easy access to in-person visits due to pandemic-related care deferral. The ability to deliver connected care in chronic diseases that requires long-term management is enhanced by artificial intelligence and virtual options of care. People with these diseases will continue to unlock opportunities for technology and consumer retail products.

Nursing must leverage the improvement in efficient and effective communication with individual patients and populations of patients for whom they care. Nursing has long recognized the need to advocate for individual patient control of the development and implementation of their plan for health and well-being. They also recognize that having simplified access to treatment options and specialty care can improve clinical outcomes and population health. Nurse informaticists are in an essential pivotal position to enhance the design and delivery of such powerful integration of data and consumer intelligence.

During COVID-19, nurse informaticists quickly rallied for the nursing team to convert to virtual learning which could be done safely. They implemented technology solutions for care delivery with iPad integration and clinical documentation that allowed COVID-19 patients to talk to their families and clinicians, that is talking to each other rather than going into patients' rooms when not necessary. The entire team presented with courage and tenacity to help lead the development of new models of patient care enabled by digital technology.

In the M Health Fairview virtual command center, during COVID-19 and now as an ongoing part of the operational leadership team reports out twice a week, technology enhancements to care and challenges for clinicians are regularly and consistently highlighted. Having a critical mass of nursing leaders, informaticists and front-line nursing workforce who understood, supported and welcomed technology as an opportunity to improve the quality and safety of nursing care was critical to success, safety and quality outcomes. This ongoing combination of factors will be critical to the success of nursing's contributions to digital transformation that improves communication, allows and empowers individuals to have more control over their care and overall improve the health of those we serve.

Electronic Documentation

Historical Review

Nursing documentation history is rich and dates back to the Crimean War with Florence Nightingale (1820–1910), the social reformer, statistician and renowned founder of nursing practice and the documentation of her findings, experience, perceptions and evidence to support recommended changes in practice (American Nursing History, n.d.). The patient's medical record began taking shape as each discipline documented in their own section, with a section specifically dedicated to medical orders and to a chart tracking of patient vital signs, which later became flowsheets. Over many decades, nursing notes progressed from end of shift summary notes, using black, blue or red ink, depending on your designated shift assignment, to highly complex and sophisticated assessments reflecting the nurses' critical thinking in assessments, interventions, planning and evaluation of patient outcomes in the form of SOAP (Subjective, Objective, Assessment and Plan) notes (circa 1968). Adapted from physician colleagues, SOAP notes were one of the very first templates nurses used to guide communication of patient care within and across disciplines.

The need to codify information and information management identified during WWII resulted in the development of computers, with the first-known devices to debut in the 1940s. As technology and computers gave birth to health informatics, circa 1974, the electronic health record (EHR) was adopted to codify patient information and improve communication within the healthcare team. Clinicians and health systems began to rely on computer and software to aid in patient care planning and decision-making (Cesnik & Kidd, 2010). The EHR provides the healthcare team with a detailed picture of the patient's progress over time, identifies early warning signs of patient changes, and improves patient safety and outcomes. While the reported root cause of many medical and medication errors was attributed to illegible handwritten medical orders and notes, the original EHR documentation reduced medication-related errors by more than 50% (American Nursing History, n.d.). The EHR now provides organizations with immense amounts and types of data which is invaluable to healthcare organizations to continue to inform and continue to improve patient care quality and safety.

The massive data available from documenting patient care is not without limitations, however. The data is limited by human input into the healthcare record. Charting by exception (CBE) or variance documentation provided the benefit of reducing the massive amounts of nursing documentation required to document variance or exception to the established 'within normal limits' parameters. Charting by exception decreased charting time, reduced redundancies in documentation and leveraged the use of well-designed flowsheets to document changes to the patient condition. Documenting using CBE reduced documentation time, returning nurses to the bedside, and also had limitations. The use of CBE required detailed protocols, initial staff training and remediation, and risk for data omission which presents the potential for legal and regulatory risk to the healthcare organization (Smith, 2002). Today, many nursing scholars and informaticists still hold firmly to the belief of the adage 'if it's not documented, it's not done.'

The Electronic Health Record of Today

The current state of nursing informatics is the result of the dedication and innovation of nursing informaticist pioneers such as Dr. Virgina Saba, PhD, RN, FAAN, FACMI, Dr. Patricia Abbott, PhD, RN, FAAN, FACMI (University of Maryland), Dr. Suzanne Bakken DNSc, RN, FAAN, FACMI (Columbia University), and Dr. Connie Delaney PhD, RN, FAAN, FACMI (University of Minnesota) (AMIA, n.d.). Comprehensive high-quality nursing documentation in the electronic healthcare record is essential to effectively contribute to the interdisciplinary plan of care, improve patient care quality, safety and outcomes. Through the EHR, nurses leverage the computer to support the nursing process, plan patient care, analyze the quality of care and provide patients with multimodal information to support self-care, well-being and shared decision-making.

Digitized and codified evidence-based content embedded into the EHR assists nurses with selecting collaborative problems, nursing diagnoses, appropriate interventions and collaborative goals and outcome criteria for patients (Carpenito-Moyet, 2004). Digital electronic patient care plans provide nurses with decision support at the point of care thereby guiding the delivery of evidence-based nursing care, improving patient care quality and safety outcomes (Gugerty & Delaney, 2009). Today, the digital care plan guidance within the EHRs integrates regulatory requirements, accreditation and quality standards, as well as professional nursing practice standards (Carpenito-Moyete, 2004). We can link policies, procedures and evidence-based resources to care plans. An example is linking drug informa-tion to medication administration records the point of care. The integrated EHR supports decision-making, safety and quality assessment.

Through the application and codification using such systems as ICD-10, RxNorm, NIC/NOC/NANDA, and other coding and tagging systems in the digital plan of care and diagnosis codes, the EHR can suggest relevant patient education and information for the nurses to select and provide patients with information sheets, videos or audio clips. Through these sys-tems, documentation of patient education, improving the health literacy of patients, engaging them in shared decision-making as part of the healthcare team, can improve patient care outcomes and safety.

The EHR documentation today is not without limitations. Nursing docu-mentation may be cumbersome, duplicative and even potentially limit the growth of critical thinking through developing an automaton or check-box mentality. The EHR is beyond data-rich; it is data massive. There is more information available to us that we have yet to fully realize how to har-ness and leverage this information to create efficiencies and improve care delivery.

The Places We Could Go

As previously stated, we are just starting to use the data available to us. Through EHR data, we are beginning to leverage patient care demograph-ics such as geographical location, age, previous hospitalizations and other psycho-social determinants of health to incorporate social determinants of health and focus on clinical decision-making, which will assist in how we plan patient care, engage public health and community resources and provide patients with the assistance they need to optimize their health lit-eracy and healthcare outcomes. For continuity of patient care the EHR can share patient care plans across healthcare systems, states and even globally. Healthcare organizations are sharing information on evidence-based stan-dards of care; we have nearly immediate access to the newest guidelines, best practices and evidence in the literature which we can integrate into patient care. Through technology such as artificial intelligence, leveraging risk factors and psycho-social determinants of health can predict patient care outcomes as related to treatment plans. Technology is enabling us to move from a primarily reactive care model for acute and chronic illness to one of preventive care in ambulatory care and community health programs to optimize healthcare for all.

Nurse Leaders and Digital Reality

The impact of digital transformation on nurse leaders and nurse executives has been as swift and substantial as it has been for nurses at the point of care and patients/consumers. Although recognition of this impact may have been catalyzed by the COVID-19 pandemic, nurse leaders report that advances in technology are here to stay (Joslin Marketing & American Organization for Nursing Leadership, 2021). Daily responsibilities include utilizing data in virtually all aspects of decision-making are essential. For example, forecasting staffing and scheduling, supply management, improving the health of populations, patient care needs and the hour-by-hour management of decisions that are required for safe patient care are all facilitated by digital information.

Competencies for point of care nurses evolve as science and technology drives new skills. This is validated as we study the work of nurses over the past century. Evolving nurse leader/nurse executive competencies also reflect advances in science (American Nurses Association). The American Organization for Nursing Leadership (AONL) competencies for nurse executives and nurse leaders have long been considered the 'brain trust' of the leadership association (Waxman et al., 2017). There are four core competency domains for nurse executives: Communication and relationship management, knowledge of the healthcare environment; Leadership; Professionalism; and Business Skills, Information Management and Technology are specifically outlined as components contained in the domain of Business Skills (American Organization for Nursing Leadership, 2015).

For nurse leaders, The AONL nurse leader (manager) competencies consist of three domains: The Science: Managing the Business; The Art: Leading the People; and The Leader Within: Creating the Leader in Yourself. Technology is a component of The Science domain (American Organization for Nursing Leadership, 2015). One could argue that since the initial articulation of the AONL competencies, digital transformation and technology have permeated through the definitions of these components. As this chapter goes to print, AONL subject matter experts are reviewing and revising the definitions of the evolving core competencies to reflect current and future practice for nurse executives/leaders, including informatics expertise.

Workforce

Nursing, as well as other healthcare professions, is facing daunting workforce challenges. The expected baby boomer retirements have begun. Nurses over the age of 65 years represent 19.0% of the RN workforce, up from 14.6% in 2017. They also comprise the largest age category. The aging of the nursing workforce is expected to continue: in a 2020 study by the National Council of State Boards of Nursing, more than one-fifth of all nurse respondents plan to retire in the next 5 years (Smiley et al., 2021).

As of this writing, the impact of COVID-19 on the nursing shortage is reaching crisis proportions. A recent letter from ANA to the US Health and Human Services secretary called for immediate action on the nursing shortage (Davis, 2021). Although the full effects of the pandemic upon the workforce are yet unknown, the psychological well-being of many caregivers (including nurses) has been severely challenged. Concern about an early exodus from the profession by pre-retirement age nurses is being expressed by many nurse leaders (Joslin Marketing & American Organization for Nursing Leadership, 2021). The latest (pre-pandemic) projection by the US Bureau of Labor Statistics indicated that Registered Nursing (RN) is among the top occupations in terms of job growth through the end of the decade. The Bureau also projects that the RN job openings each year through 2029 to be 175,900, accounting for planned retirements and attrition (Bureau of Labor Statistics). These projections do not include the effect of the pandemic upon early retirement or attrition and will need to be carefully monitored for future workforce needs. The importance of immediate information related to the workforce from all healthcare delivery settings, regionally, nationally and globally, cannot be overstated. The comprehensive data on supply and demand for current and future workforce needs is paramount to ensuring the health and safety of our communities. Nurse leaders, who are responsible for the delivery of care, must have access to the information as well as have the competencies to evaluate, plan, implement and assess the outcomes of their work in this arena.

The COVID-19 pandemic initiated a number of innovations that, in some cases, resulted in changes to the 'rules.' One widely utilized technology, telehealth, was able to be implemented rapidly due to the CMS Emergency Declaration Blanket Waivers that resulted in increased access and facilitated care. Another waiver that was granted and was enthusiastically received by providers and caregivers included the provisions related to documentation of nursing care plans and verbal orders (Centers for Medicare and Medicaid

Services, 2020). This allowed for more time to be spent in essential functions (direct patient care) versus documentation. These are just two of many examples. COVID-19 has been cited as a 'catalyst' for transformation in healthcare, as well as virtually every other sector (Atalla, 2021). As we look to the future when the COVID-19 crisis abates, the question remains as to whether and what innovations will and should continue. There are numerous factors to consider and outcomes to be studied. However, it is apparent that the speed of implementation and the rapid adoption of innovations were substantial and will propel us forward towards true digital transformation.

Call to Action

For successful and sustained digital transformation in healthcare that is focused on the health of our patients and communities, nurses will be integral to the process. This will require nurses and nurse leaders to be champions, a role that may not be within one's 'comfort zone.' Active promotion of appropriate digital tools to enhance care and promote health will be required, as will the personal competency of critical evaluation of utility from the perspective of clinician/caregiver and patient/consumer. To be successful, this change in perspective must be incorporated in formal education, beginning at the pre-licensure level and continuing through all levels. Nurse researchers, in particular, have a mandate to determine if the science driving digital transformation is having the desired outcome for both the nurses and the population. Nurses in practice will need to be given the opportunity to learn new skills. Nurse leaders in all settings will be required to become competent personally, as well as plan for the deployment of technology and education for their team. Advocacy for resources will be pivotal in this work.

References

American Nurses Association. (n.d.) [online]. Available at: https://www.nursingwo rld.org/globalassets/practiceandpolicy/nursing-excellence/ana-position-state-ments-secure/nursing-practice/professional-role-competence.pdf (Accessed September 23 2021).

American Organization for Nursing Leadership. (2015a). *Nurse executive competencies* [online]. Available at: https://www.aonl.org/system/files/media/file/2019/06/nec.pdf (Accessed September 16 2021).

American Organization for Nursing Leadership. (2015b). *Nurse manager competencies* [online]. Available at: https://www.aonl.org/system/files/media/file/2019/06/nurse-manager-competencies.pdf (Accessed September 12 2021).

Atalla, G. (2021, January). *Embracing digital: is COVID-19 the catalyst for lasting change?* [online]. Available at: https://www.ey.com/en_us/government-public-sector/embracing-digital-is-covid-19-the-catalyst-for-lasting-change (Accessed September 15 2021).

Bureau of Labor Statistics, & U.S. Department of Labor. (2021, August). *Occupational outlook handbook*, Registered Nurses [online]. Available at: https://www.bls.gov/ooh/healthcare/registered-nurses.htm (Accessed September 23 2021).

Business Wire. (2021, July). *United States healthcare consumerism growth opportunities: analyzing SDOH data to improve patient outcomes and empower consumers* [online]. Available at: https://www.businesswire.com/news/home/20210730005181/en/United-States-Healthcare-Consumerism-Growth-Opportunities-Analyzing-SDOH-Data-to-Improve-Patient-Outcomes-and-Empower-Consumers---ResearchAndMarkets.com (Accessed September 18 2021).

Carpenito-Moyet, L. J. (2004). *Nursing care plans & documentation. [electronic resource]: Nursing diagnoses and collaborative problems.* 4th ed. Philadelphia, PA: Lippincott Williams & Wilkins.

Centers for Medicare and Medicaid Services. (2020, March). *COVID-19 emergency declaration blanket waivers for health care providers* [online]. Available at: https://www.cms.gov/files/document/covid19-emergency-declaration-health-care-providers-fact-sheet.pdf (Accessed September 23 2021).

Cesnik, B., & Kidd, M. R. (2010). History of health informatics: a global perspective. *Studies in Health Technology and Informatics*, 151, pp.3–8.

Davis, C. (2021, September). *ANA calls for the nurse staffing shortage to be declared a national crisis* [online]. Available at: https://www.healthleadersmedia.com/nursing/ana-calls-nurse-staffing-shortage-be-declared-national-crisis (Accessed September 25 2021).

Gugerty, B., & Delaney, C. (2009, August). *Technology informatics guiding educational reform (TIGER).* TIGER Informatics Competencies Collaborative (TICC) Final Report [online]. Available at: http://tigercompetencies.pbworks.com/f/TICC_Final.pdf (Accessed September 23 2021).

Jones, G. L., Peter, Z., Rutter, Dr. K.-A., & Somauroo, A. (2019, June). *Promoting an overdue digital transformation in healthcare* [online]. Available at: https://www.mckinsey.com/industries/healthcare-systems-and-services/our-insights/promoting-an-overdue-digital-transformation-in-healthcare (Accessed September 19 2021).

Joslin Marketing, & AONL. (2021). *Nursing leadership COVID-19 insight longitudinal study* [online]. Available at: https://www.aonl.org/system/files/media/file/2021/03/PublicJoslin2.0.pdf. (Accessed September 23 2021).

Nursing Documentation Historical Review. (n.d.). *American nursing history* [online]. Available at: https://www.americannursinghistory.org/documentation (Accessed August 28 2021).

Nursing Informatics Innovators (AMIA). [online]. Available at: https://amia.org/community/working-groups/nursing-informatics/nursing-informatics-innovators (Accessed September 23 2021).

Research and Markets. (2021, July). *United States healthcare consumerism growth opportunities* [online]. Available at: https://www.researchandmarkets.com/reports/5387763/united-states-healthcare-consumerism-growth?utm_source=BW&utm_medium=PressRelease&utm_code=95x6vn&utm_campaign=1567915+-+United+States+Healthcare+Consumerism+Growth+Opportunities%3a+Analyzing+SDOH+Data+to+Improve+Patient+Outcomes+and+Empower+Consumers&utm_exec=cari18prd (Accessed September 3 2021).

Smiley, R. A., Ruttinger, C., Oliveira, C. M., Reneau, K. A., Silvestre, J. H., & Alexander, M. (2021, April). *The 2020 national nursing workforce survey* [online]. Available at: https://www.journalofnursingregulation.com/article/S2155-8256(21)00027-2/fulltext#secst0010 (Accessed September 23 2021).

Smith, L. S. (2002, September). *How to chart by exception: Nursing2021.* Nursing 2021 [online]. Available at: https://journals.lww.com/nursing/fulltext/2002/09000/how_to_chart_by_exception.18.aspx (Accessed September 19 2021).

Takyar, A. (n.d.). *The impact of digital transformation in healthcare* [online]. Available at: https://www.leewayhertz.com/digital-transformation-in-healthcare/ (Accessed September 11 2021).

Waxman, K. T., Roussel, L., Herrin-Griffith, D., & D'Alfonso, J. (2017, April). *The AONE nurse executive competencies: 12 Years later* [online]. Available at: https://www.sciencedirect.com/science/article/abs/pii/S1541461216302555 (Accessed September 23 2021).

Chapter 6

Engage the People: Health Informatics and Personal Health Management

Anne Moen, Amy Cramer and Catherine Chronaki

Contents

Introduction

The starting point and premise for this chapter are the significant, unmet needs within our populations and the opportunity for novel digital health solutions to support everyday health management (Moen and Brennan, 2005; Zayas-Cabán, 2012; Casper et al., 2016). Although there is broad consensus that the patient's needs should drive demand, more often other

DOI: 10.4324/9781003054849-6

considerations take precedence including sustainability of the health system, workforce shortage, fear of the unknown, market regulation, monetization of data or shifting of traditional role expectations (van Riel et al., 2019). However, from the individual's perspective, several factors can influence health decisions, such as knowledge, interests and capabilities, priorities and preferences for participation (Brennan & Casper, 2015). These dynamics underlie everyday health choices that carry shorter- and longer-term consequences for an individual's health and wellness. We know that most households have an '*informal, Chief Health Officer*' (CHO) that pays attention to relevant health matters, manages important interactions around health and wellness, and keeps track of information relative to daily living, health situation, goals and preferences in the household (Moen & Brennan, 2005). It is essential to equip these informal CHOs with the right digital tools to transparently collect and complement the pertinent information, employ analytics and make decisions.

CHOs are health consumers that appreciate convenience. For example, the CHOs are responsible for keeping a comprehensive overview of the health and illness of family members, for identifying price estimates and flexible payment options, and for electronically scheduling appointments available in most health systems. However, healthcare systems often fall short in meeting such expectations and that is to the detriment of safeguarding the health of the population. All too often, individuals experience limited access to their own information, which is dispersed across diverse actors in health and care. As it stands today, coordinating content from multiple sources and health facilities is stressing and time-demanding for the CHO since the information support offered by traditional health systems is quite limited. Systematic activation, along with opportunities for engagement, prevention and early intervention can encourage participation and self-management for an individual to maintain functional abilities, dignity and to thrive (Østensen et al., 2016).

Despite some efforts and achievements to improve access to personal, health-related information, opportunities to actively use this information to navigate the health system and fully comprehend/understand the implications of one's data represents a challenge for almost everyone. One limiting factor is the uniform and consistent adoption of interoperability standards allowing for the seamless exchange, harmonization and use of data. Data can be exchanged instantly for many other daily uses, such as the electronic exchange of money. Deposits, withdrawals and purchases can all be made by electronically exchanging money, which is data. This is possible because the financial industry agreed on their standards when building their systems for electronic transactions. Standards provide the framework for semantic interoperability, i.e., agreed-upon understanding of what the data represents, and structural interoperability, i.e., agreed-upon format for how the data is exchanged.

Nowadays, with the emergence of the HL7® Fast Healthcare Interoperability Resources (FHIR®) standard, healthcare data is moving towards a universally agreed-upon interoperability standard. This standard allows for data to be electronically exchanged in real-time with both semantic and structural integrity as well as data security. HL7 FHIR® is rapidly being adopted by large and small tech vendors, regulatory agencies, third-party payers and pharmaceutical companies, among many others (HL7, 2019). HL7 FHIR® powers systems that expose an interface to patients, such as Apple's Health Kit and the International Patient Summary (IPS) that facilitate access to key health and wellness information. HL7 FHIR® is changing the way healthcare data can be received and reviewed. However, there are still very few tools and services that are designed or deployed to actively engage and empower citizens to be 'on top of' their own health information and manage all this information in collaboration with their care provider(s) at different levels of care, health systems and organizations. Health data analytics in general do not observe data quality and interoperability standards, leaving important ethical issues unresolved (Leung et al., 2019).

The 'Inverse Care Law' proposed by Hart (1971) still applies in today's digital reality. This is to say that the availability and productive use of digital health tools varies inversely with the actual needs. Thus, our current state is one in which access to and adoption of digital tools underscores persistent disparities in healthcare. Patient information remains fragmented, and chains of health and care activity are most often broken, largely due to technical and structural obstacles. These include limited or partial access to health records systems, lack of interoperability and little opportunity to actively select or use information for relevant, everyday purposes (Wibe et al., 2015; Hibbard & Greene, 2013). We observe that providers and health systems increasingly offer access via dedicated, secure portals as a service to their members and patients. The individual can manually enter information into specific applications of personal choice or keep the information as paper files—more or less organized. This situation leads to a mix of data in incompatible formats ranging from access to subsets of personal health information in digital form, image sets in digital media and digital snippets of exchanges and data in static paper documents subject to the person's choice.

This situation calls for ad-hoc, time-consuming and non-scaling strategies in navigating and comprehending the plethora of disconnected information, often without quality control or reliable guidance, thereby creating confusion leading to misinformation.

Fragmented or unavailable health information can create a significant risk of errors (Coiera et al., 2011), unintended adverse events or even premature deaths (Helse- og omsorgsdepartementet, 2014). In the area of medication management, the magnitude of the challenge for the individual and society are demonstrated by the World Health Organization's (WHO) reporting that more than 50% of all medicines are prescribed, dispensed or sold inappropriately worldwide (WHO, 2002). In fact, estimates suggest that as many as 125.000 premature deaths are caused each year in the United States (US) (Martin et al., 2005), and around 200,000 premature deaths annually in Europe due to poor adherence to treatment (OECD, 2020). In addition to the personal cost and burden, these challenges with inappropriate medication use and adherence to treatment carry a high societal cost that puts a significant burden on healthcare systems (Cutler et al., 2018). Even minor improvements could present great potential for personal gains and societal improvement, ensuring health and well-being for all, aligned with the United Nations SDG3 'ensure healthy lives and promote wellbeing at all ages' (United Nations, 2015). Thus, there is significant untapped potential for nursing and health informatics to mobilize and support prevention and early intervention, thereby avoiding costly treatments and improving our populations' health. All these goals remain at the core of our nursing profession, service and research.

Obvious Paradox – Opportunities for Health Informatics

Health information systems in use today seek to optimize health systems operations and support health providers in making operational planning. At the same time, current health systems research focuses on the resilience of health organizations and health systems employing machine learning and analytics (Ozcan, 2017). However, many health informatics solutions fall short of consumer convenience, as there are very few tools available for wider availability that facilitate the active use of health information by individuals. The rapid shift to virtual communication for many care and treatment purposes has uncovered the importance of active use of personal health information. To receive the full benefit of such applications, it becomes increasingly important for the individual to have good digital skills and appropriate health literacy for comprehension of cues, concerns and consequences (Sørensen et al., 2012).

The growing use of digital tools currently offers little support for holistic personal health information management, as overseen by a household's self-appointed CHO (Moen, 2007). Studies of these activities demonstrate diverse, sophisticated, robust strategies to differentiate and handle the already fragmented health information for personal purposes (Moen & Brennan, 2005), including:

- *Just-in-time*, i.e., information and/or artifacts are with me at most times
- *Just-at-hand*, i.e., information and/or artifacts are visible or stored in readily accessible, highly familiar locations in a household
- *Just-in-case*, i.e., information and/or artifacts, either personal health files or general health information resources, are kept away, but are easily retrievable
- *Just-because*, i.e., information and/or artifacts of temporal relevance, kept in the household until storage strategy is assigned.

These strategies illustrate appraisal of the information, the anticipation of need, balancing confidentiality and privacy of the information against an interest in adding or sharing information, ensuring continuity and avoiding fragmentation of health data (Moen & Brennan, 2005). The specifics of these strategies can be very personal, sophisticated and robust for self-management in the 'care-between-care' periods or in guiding 'inter-visit' care actions (Brennan & Casper, 2015). Therefore, understanding data management strategies are key to bridging any gaps that may happen when using both person-generated data with those of the provider(s).

Going forward we need to systematically alleviate what we think is an obvious paradox: Despite interest in and expectations for personal health management, there are few comprehensive digital solutions to support everyday activities by individuals and in collaboration with the household's CHO. What is needed is to create tools that enable us to collect, compile, curate and integrate health information from multiple institutions, services and systems. Then, we have the opportunity to share consolidated parts of this information with providers, significantly contributing to continuity in ongoing care and treatment. New digital health services that support and offer a good overview of health information with an understanding of its implications, if successfully deployed at scale will come with opportunities to engage, improve user experience and empower the individual (Moen, 2018).

The European Union (EU) General Data Protection Regulation on Data Portability (GDPR) (European Parliament, 2016) and national laws, like the Norwegian Patient Act (Helse- og omsorgsdepartementet, 2001), state that it is every citizen's right to a digital copy of their data and that includes their health information. Similarly, the US 21st Century Cure Act includes measures to prevent and prohibit information blocking (Health Human Services, 2020). These EU and US regulations create a fertile environment for digital services that can enable and empower participation and management of personal health information for self or family members for everyday purposes, while enabling collaboration with health providers and informed decision making. In this context, HL7 FHIR® is the de facto standard for providing uniform and harmonized access to the disparate sources of health data.

In Europe, research and development activities have grappled with the challenges of mobility, and orientation in new contexts, especially for navigation in health and care (Chronaki et al., 2017). Additionally, in the European context of cross-border healthcare services, the *'International Patient Summary'* (IPS) emerged to support patient safety and informed care provision in situations for unplanned care in another country (Heitman et al., 2018; Kay et al., 2020). The next section presents examples of solutions seeking to meet consumers' expectations for ease of access to their health information and for usefulness in managing specific health needs.

Case Examples: Patient-Centered Digital Tools and Services

Two case examples illustrate our observations on the changes coming with usable digital services for the least supported resources in healthcare: *the person*, in the role of patient or family member, or informal caregiver. These examples build on data and information and point to opportunities for the improvement of healthcare experiences. Change and responsible innovation via emerging digital services provide convenience for the individual and support patient safety while respecting the person's preferred level of engagement.

Personal Use of Wearables, Sensors and IoT for Safety in Ambient Active Living

The pervasiveness of mobile sensors and wide-spread adoption of wearable devices (Internet of Things devices (IoT)), and growing numbers and types of implants used for treatment and care, all generate massive amounts of data that are accumulated in many formats and used for a broad set of health activities. Sensors and IoT devices provide data that can offer insights into human processes, as well as the activities in the environment, including health and wellness-related activities in the home.

As an example, the Norwegian government prepared the whitepaper 'Innovation in Care' (Helse- og omsorgsdepartementet, 2011) a decade ago, and recently launched the program 'Leve Hele Livet' (A full life—all your life—A Quality Reform for Older Persons) (Helse - og omsorgsdepartementet, 2018) to accelerate the uptake of *Best Practices for Age Friendly Communities* (KS, 2021). The overall goal is to stimulate improvements in areas of early intervention, prevention and cooperation through a program that focuses on nutrition, sound medication management and providing for safe physical environments and digital services. Increasingly offered as part of the community healthcare service, we see several types of services and digital tools emerging to enable aging-in-place, and in age-friendly and safe environments (Helse- og omsorgsdepartementet, 2018). Therefore, several approaches have been explored in terms of feasibility, safety and attractiveness. These include:

1) Physical environment optimization; either in the house, e.g., new or retrofitting with good contrast, overview, light, door-video or outdoor, e.g., rails, sturdy surface, accessibility to ensure control and safety
2) Senso-based surveillance, which can be seen as 'passive monitoring' of activities in the home environment or with the person while mobile, including GPS (global positioning system), safe home environment ('stove watch,' light sensors), personal safety (fall prevention in particular)
3) Engagements tools, like networking and personal enjoyment, or video-based health consultations to stimulate active contributions for prevention, early intervention or rehabilitation for a better health and life experience
4) Tools for mental, physical or social stimulation and recall, like social robots named Paro or Pepper, or outdoor garden (Dahlkvist et al., 2020) or 'traveling' via 'street-view' maps of a chosen, well-known surroundings
5) Support for informal caregivers, tools for targeted purpose- or condition-specific information, sharing and preparing for special roles or responsibilities, e.g., demonstration of tools used in the home, or preparing for challenging care experiences (Janson et al., 2020a).

GATEKEEPER (www.gatekeeper-project.eu), building on results of its pre-decessor project ActiveAge (Fico et al., 2018), is a European multicentric, large-scale pilot on 'Smart Living Environments' connecting healthcare providers, businesses, entrepreneurs, elderly citizens and their communities. The aim is to ensure healthier, independent lives for the aging populations, improving the quality of life of citizens while demonstrating efficiency gains in health and care delivery across Europe. Development efforts focus on creating an open, trust-based arena for matching ideas, technologies, user needs and processes. The standardization strategy is an actionable, agile part of GATEKEEPER as it aims at creating a digital health service ecosys-tem powered by data analytics. The HL7 FHIR® Implementation Guide (IG) of GATEKEEPER has been created to accelerate the integration of reusable IoT devices, sensor components and health analytics into services offered across Europe. Notably, mentoring is an integral part of the service redesign and consistently employs the HL7 FHIR® IG to align new services to the existing portfolio. In this sense, GATEKEEPER can help advance the quality and consistency of health data, driving better algorithms for data analytics. Besides this purely technical perspective, one should not lose sight of bio-ethics, particularly in relation to data analytics and Artificial Intelligence (AI). The data used to fuel analytics should be high quality, offer no bias and be able to explain the reason for a decision or the outcome, i.e., explainable AI (European Commission, 2021). Building trust is essential and a role that is well suited to nursing. Nurses should be proficient users of systems, such as GATEKEEPER and X-eHealth, to advise, direct and educate patients, along the lines of 'My data—My Decision—Our e-Power' (Chronaki et al., 2017).

Personal Collection, Management and Custodianship of Personal Health Information

Interoperability and health informatics standards make access between dis-parate (individual and provider) systems possible. Privacy and security con-cerns, with technical, organizational and interoperability standards become important drivers for new paradigms.

Standards make data available, leading to the development of curated information summaries, like the IPS. Such summary documents can include allergies, medications, problem list and discharge summary (Chronaki et al., 2015). The IPS presents curated, relevant information for patient and pro-vider-mediated exchange. Therefore, should an urgent need or unplanned care episode occur, when in another country or health system, the person and their new health providers can start from a patient summary fit for the purpose of sharing critical health information. The technical feasibility of the IPS concept has been successfully tested, and also identifying limitations of transforming clinically equivalent sections used in Europe to those used in the US (Estelrich et al., 2015, Heitmann et al., 2018). Therefore, the EU-funded X-eHealth project set out to develop the 'European EHR-exchange Format' (EHRxF) that would add new guidance and detailed specifications for patient summaries, prescription, laboratory and imaging results (Bonacina et al., 2021). After the episode of care, a person can receive a discharge summary or encounter report for future use in support of continuity of care. Privacy and security concerns, with technical, organizational and interoperability standards come as important drivers. To reap benefits, human factors and professional accountability are important for uptake and to gradually improve the summary documents. x-eHealth strives to stimulate interconnected Communities of Practice that benefit from the EHRxF.

Personal experience, capacity and digital health literacy are important to fully understand and appreciate the potential of these new digital services. Further advancement is expected as co-creation processes starting from the IPS can bring patients, health professionals and informal caregivers together. Co-creation and participatory design facilitate the usability and usefulness of a solution. This approach is especially important in designing visualizations that are understandable and actionable, information promoting, and that gain active engagement across groups with variable degrees of digital health literacy skills (Arcia et al., 2016). To maintain trust and data integrity of the contributions from patients and providers, it is essential to clarify stewardship when sharing, interpreting and complementing health information. With summary documents, we would argue that they are essential for continuity of care and treatment, as well as to support mobility and activities in different contexts of care. Increasingly digitally and health literate persons can contribute to a stronger basis for the decision and everyday health choices. Ultimately, the key to creating an environment for responsible innovation is remembering that innovation travels at the speed of trust.

The *CAPABLE* project is another example, where the goal is a digital solution for active, personal health information management (Hurlen & Moen, 2019). The starting point is also with areas where information elements are at the core in the IPS. *CAPABLE* comes with an explicit focus on user engagement and empowerment through a tool designed for individuals, not for the providers or health system owners. As such, *CAPABLE* seeks to balance the complex demands for functionality, comprehension and easy-to-use solutions with usability and usefulness. Therefore, the solution should seek to be accessible with understandable content, high performance, and guarantee security, privacy, and trustworthiness (Janson et al., 2020b). Following this, a user of *CAPABLE* can copy, curate and add—*not substitute or alter*—health data from providers, and add personal observations. Importantly, the individual can choose to share their data with health providers when and for as long as they feel this is needed. Users will have the opportunity to report errors and correct information on what matters to them starting with visits, medications and their effects. The design of *CAPABLE* is driven by a commitment to equip and empower citizens with understandable and actionable health information that meets their personal needs. The system will be available as an affordable and effective service where the personal health information they wish to collect, complement and control can be safely stored. As such, the solution provides universally designed, functional digital tools where a person can handle personal health matters, as the personal or household's CHO already does with more rudimentary, non-scaling tools.

Building from the *IPS*, *CAPABLE* and other citizen-centered solutions, we will continue to create a new tool *G-Lens*, which aims to offer novel personal health information improvement for many users, particularly those who take numerous medications to control complex health conditions. G-Lens will introduce digital services based on a focusing mechanism, taking components in the IPS to feed rules that will highlight information in the medicinal product information—ePI (electronic product information by EMA, 2021). The ePI can make approved information from a regulator about medication in use more accessible, increase understanding and actionability by patients and health professionals (Moen et al., 2021). The goal is to create a more convenient health experience, where citizens are confident, active and responsive in personal health management, reduce fragmentation and encourage safe use of medicines for better health outcomes and quality of life.

The Expanded Nurses' Role

Nursing programs should prepare the nurses of the future to play the role of health information technology brokers (Matney et al., 2015). As digital health solutions penetrate our societies, nurses will continue to significantly impact their patients' health through multiple avenues and new roles as that of a digital technology mediator and broker. Trust is paramount to winning the adoption of these new patient-centered, digital solutions, and nurses are perfectly poised to lead this paradigm shift in healthcare. In turn, learning how to use these new digital tools and their underlying technologies, to the extent that they are able to teach safe use to their patients, represents a steep learning curve. Nurse informaticists need to be ready to support nurses in this undertaking in all settings: classrooms, simulation labs and in care delivery settings like hospitals and home. Importantly, nurses will need to take on the tasks of helping people to manage the data generated by their new digital solutions.

For nursing, collaboration with the patient and their family members/informal caregiver and the family's CHO will involve introducing these new digital tools as part of their care plan. Mentoring to become expert users will strengthen their capacity for everyday self-care and self-management by being competent custodians of their data. Digital Services, functionality and qualities that add convenience and control for the patient can also reduce pressure on nurses, primary care providers as well as specialized health services, and help comprehension or sense-making of health and care situations when literarily 'bombarded' with suggestions and information of different origin and quality. In this context, attention to updated information from an IPS and relevant 'Observations of Daily Living' can support quite specific but contextual and personal comprehension of cues and concerns to follow up ongoing treatment and therapies for best possible outcomes. Digital health tools create value and strengthen health information management, collaboration and service coordination, based on sharing of the information at the user's discretion. Active engagement and collaboration in digital tools that support diverse information needs for self-care, treatment and self-management will add to the nurse's role that of a trusted advisor for health information technology.

Discussion

Overcoming Hart's inverse law paradox on the high interest in digital services, but the reality being a lack of comprehensive digital solutions to support the person at their chosen site of activity continues to be a challenge. Usable digital services are needed to equip the most important but least supported resources in healthcare—*the person*, as patient, informal caregiver or family member, with opportunities to use their health information at their discretion and convenience. If approached with respect, dignity and care for the person, such activities represent an untapped potential for value creation and improvement of healthcare experiences, with innovation delivered via novel, digital health services.

Delivery of digital health services where health information is available can engage, equip and empower the individual, allowing meaningful participation and shared decision making. Liberating the information and creating tools for active use of personal health information can redress the traditional asymmetrical relationships in healthcare, where patients are regarded as mostly passive recipients. Tools powered by analytics can shift the balance and result in concrete benefits for the individual and the health system as a whole. In these information processes the goal is that the users can (1) access, understand and apply information, (2) complement information with personal, relevant comments (annotate/update) as they like/need, (3) collaborate with trusted partners and the healthcare team and (4) preserve control over personal health information by choosing 'what to share, with whom, and for how long' (Moen, 2018). These are central notions in the Digital Health Compass created by eStandards, the European initiative that developed a roadmap for standardization to support the large-scale deployment of digital health services (Chronaki et al., 2017).

The full benefits experienced convenience and value proposition, usable digital services to mobilize the least supported resources in healthcare; *the person themselves*, as patients or family members, represents an untapped potential for change and innovation via novel digital health services. Purposeful, specific digital solutions that responsibly balance transparency, safety, trust, security and privacy with increasing engagement, participation and empowerment can make a significant difference in the ongoing digital transformation in healthcare systems.

Summary

Patients and their families represent the most important participants in healthcare. They represent an undervalued resource that, if mobilized, could significantly change the interactions and improve the health and wellness of the individual (Leung et al., 2019). Well-designed digital solutions can deliver much-needed tools with benefits for all. Engagement, active participation and empowerment can shift our societies to wellness and prevention-oriented, healthcare systems with quality-of-life gains and significant economic benefits. To achieve the full advantage of a digitally transformed healthcare system, people must become digitally literate. Nursing is positioned to play the role of technology mentors and advocates to overcome the digital literacy gap and to gain trust in the applications. Literacy skills are fundamental to trust and being able to control with whom one shares their information and for how long. Digital skills and efforts to advance health literacy to comprehend cues or concerns and monitor contextual and personal health issues become a priority. Nurses are key to this transformation.

Usable, elegant tools for citizen engagement, as illustrated in the case studies presented, can help redress the traditional asymmetrical relationships in healthcare, with patients as mostly passive recipients. Future service innovation can enable transformational change by offering novel opportunities to collect, complement and curate information for personal use. Untapping the potential of these new digital technologies to alleviate unmet needs with nurses as digital mentors can help people effectively handle the health and wellness challenges they face on a daily basis.

References

Arcia, A., Suero-Tejeda, N., Bales, M. E., Merril, J. A. & Yoon, S. (2016). Sometimes more is more: Iterative participatory design of infographics for engagement of community members with varying levels of health literacy. *Journal of the American Medical Informatics Association*, 23, pp.174–183.

Bonacina, S., Koch, S., Meneses, I., & Chronaki, C. (2021) Can the European EHR exchange format support shared decision making and citizen-driven health science? *Studies in Health Technology and Informatics*, 281, pp.1056–1060. https://doi.org/10.3233/shti210346

Brennan, P. F., & Casper, G. R. (2015). Observing health in everyday living: ODLs and the care-between-the-care. *Personal and Ubiquitous Computing*, 11;19(1), pp.3–8.

Casper, G. R., Brennan, P. F., Smith, C. A., Werner, N. E., & He, Y. (2016). Health @ Home moves all about the house. *Studies in Health Technology and Informatics*, 216, pp.842–846. PMID: 26262170.

Chronaki, C., Moen, A., Stroetmann, V., Vander Stichele, R., Romero Gutierrez, A., Ehrler, F., & Park, H-A. (2015). *Human aspects of eHealth interoperability in the transatlantic setting*. Madrid, Spain: MIE.

Chronaki, C., Stegwee, R., & Moen, A. (2017). In search of a digital health compass to navigate the health system. *Studies in Health Technology and Informatics*, 245, pp.30–34.

Coiera, E., Aarts, J. & Kulikowski, C. (2011). The dangerous decade. *Journal of American Medical Informatics Association*, 19(1), pp.2–5.

Cutler, R. L., & Fernandez- Llimos, F., Frommer, M., Benrimoj, C., & Garcia-Cardenas, V. (2018). Economic impact of medication non-adherence by disease groups: A systematic review. *BMJ Open*, 8, p.e016982.

Dahlkvist, E., Engström, M., & Nilsson, A. (2020). Residents' use and perceptions of residential care facility gardens: A behaviour mapping and conversation study. *International Journal of Older People Nursing*, 15(1), p.e12283. https://doi.org/10.1111/opn.12283

Estelrich, A., Chronaki, C., Cangioli, G., & Melgara, M. (2015). Converging patient summaries: Finding the common denominator between the European patient summary and the US-based continuity of care document. In Proceedings of IHIC 2015, Prague.

European Commission. (2021). *Communication on fostering a European approach to artificial intelligence.* Available at: https://digital-strategy.ec.europa.eu/en/library/communication-fostering-european-approach-artificial-intelligence (Accessed September 25 2021).

European Medicines Agency (EMA). (2021). *Product information requirements* [Online]. Available at: https://www.ema.europa.eu/en/human-regulatory/marketing-authorisation/product-information-requirements (Accessed September 22 2021).

European Parliament. (2016). REGULATION (EU) 2016/679 on processing of personal data and on the free movement of such data.

Fico, G. et al. (2018) Co-creating with consumers and stakeholders to understand the benefit of internet of things in smart living environments for ageing well: The approach adopted in the Madrid deployment site of the ACTIVAGE large scale pilot. In H. Eskola, O. Väisänen, J. Viik, J. Hyttinen, eds., EMBEC & NBC 2017. IFMBE Proceedings, vol 65. Singapore: Springer. https://doi.org/10.1007/978-981-10-5122-7_272

Hart J. T. (1971). The inverse care law. *The Lancet*, 297(7696, 27), pp.405–412.

Health and Human Services. (2020). 21st Century cures act: Interoperability, information blocking, and the ONC health IT certification program. *Federal Register: Daily Journal of the US Government*, May 11.

Heitmann, K. U., Cangioli, G., Melgara, M., & Chronaki, C. (2018). Interoperability assets for patient summary components: A gap analysis. *Studies in Health Technology and Informatics*, 247, pp.700–704. PMID: 29678051.

Helse- og omsorgsdepartementet (2001). *Lov om pasient- og brukerrettigheter,* §5 ff. Available at: https://lovdata.no/dokument/NL/lov/1999-07-02-63/KAPITTEL_6#%C2%A75-1

Helse – og omsorgsdepartementet (2011). *Innovasjon i Omsorg.* NOU2011:11. Oslo.

Helse- og omsorgsdepartementet (2014). Legemiddelmeldingen, Riktig bruk - bedre helse. *Meld. St.,* 28(2014-2015), Oslo.

Helse – og omsorgsdepartementet (2018). A full life–all your life: A quality reform for older persons. *Melding til Stortinget* 15(2017–2018), Oslo.

Hibbards, J. H., & Greene, J. (2013). What the evidence shows about patient activation: Better health outcomes and care experiences; fewer data on costs. *Health Affairs*, 32(2), pp.207–214. https://doi.org/10.1377/hlthaff.2012.1061

HL7. (2019). *Fast healthcare interoperabilty resources* [Online]. Available at: https://www.hl7.org/fhir/ (Accessed September 21, 2021).

Hurlen, P., & Moen, A. (2019). Preserved in translation. *HL7 Newsletter 09*, June 2019.

Janson, A. L., Moen, A., & Fuglerud, K. S. (2020a). Design of the capable health empowerment tool: Citizens' needs and expectations. *Studies in Health Technology and Informatics*, 270, pp.926–930.

Janson, A. L., Moen, A., & Lunde, L. (2020b). En avatar som brobygger: Fra forskningsfunn til pårørendestøtte. In *Sykepleie på nye måter*. E-helsekonferansen 2020. Oslo: Norsk Sykepleierforbund.

Kay, S., Cangioli, G., & Nusbaum, M. (2020) The international patient summary standard and the extensibility requirement. *Studies in Health Technology and Informatics*, 4(273), pp.54–62. https://doi.org/10.3233/SHTI200615. PMID: 33087592

KS. (2021). *Aldersvennlige Lokalsamfunn (Age friendly communities)*. Available at: https://www.ks.no/fagomrader/velferd/aldersvennlige-lokalsamfunn/ (Accessed September 23, 2021).

Leung, K., Lu-McLean, D., Kuziemsky, C., Booth, R. G., Collins Rossetti, S, Borycki, E., & Strudwick, G. (2019). Using patient and family engagement strategies to improve outcomes of health information technology initiatives: Scoping review. *Journal of Medical Internet Research*, 21(10), p.e14683. https://doi.org/10.2196/14683

Martin, L. R., Williams, S. L., Haskard, K. B., & Dimatteo, M. R. (2005). The challenge of patient adherence. *Therapeutics and Clinical Risk Management*, 3, pp.189–199.

Matney, S., Avant, K., & Staggers, N. (2015). Toward an understanding of wisdom in nursing. *OJIN: The Online Journal of Issues in Nursing*, 21(1), p.9. https://doi.org/10.3912/OJIN.Vol21No01PPT02. PMID: 27853292.

Moen, A. (2007). Personal health information management. In W. Jones, & J. Teevan, eds., *Personal information management*. Seattle and London: University of Washington Press.

Moen, A. (2018). Citizens and health data: Untapped resource for telehealth. *Studies in Health Technology and Informatics*, 254, pp.63–69, IOS Press.

Moen, A., & Brennan, P. F. (2005). Health@Home: The work of health information management in the household (HIMH): Implications for consumer health informatics (CHI) innovations. *Journal of American Medical Informatics Association*, 12, pp.648–56.

Moen, A., Chronaki, C., Govani, A., Stichele, R. V., Hurlen, P. & Ingvar, G. (2021). G-Lens to focus medication information: Opportunities with structured ePI standard. In Workshop, MIE2021, Athens.

Organization for Economic Co-operation and Development (OECD), & European Union. (2020). *Health at a glance: Europe 2020: State of health in the EU cycle*. Paris: OECD Publishing. https://doi.org/10.1787/82129230-en (Accessed August 15 2021).

Østensen, E., Gjevjon, E. R., Øderud, T., & Moen, A. (2016). Introducing technology for thriving in residential long-term care. *Journal of Nursing Scholarship*, 49(1), pp.44–53.

Ozcan, Y. A. (2017). *Analytics and decision support in health care operations management*. 3rd ed. Jossey-Bass. ISBN: 978-1-119-21981-1.

Sørensen, K., Van den Broucke, S., Fullam, J., Doyle, G., Pelikan, J., Slonska, Z., Brand, H., & (HLS-EU) Consortium Health Literacy Project European. (2012). Health literacy and public health: A systematic review and integration of definitions and models. *BMC Public Health*, 12(1), p.80.

United Nations. (2015) *UN sustainable development goals*. United Nations. Available at: https://sdgs.un.org/goals and https://www.un.org/sustainabledevelopment/health/ (Accessed 21 September 2021).

van Riel, P. L. C. M., Zuidema, R. M., Vogel, C., & Rongen-van Dartel, S. A. (2019). Patient self-management and tracking: A European experience. *Rheumatic Disease Clinics of North America*, 45(2), pp.187–195. https://doi.org/10.1016/j.rdc.2019.01.008. PMID: 30952392

WHO. (2002). Promoting rational use of medicines: Core components. *WHO policy perspectives on medicine*. Geneva. https://apps.who.int/iris/bitstream/handle/10665/67438/WHO_EDM_2002.3.pdf

Wibe, T., Ekstedt, M., & Hellesø, R. (2015). Information practices of health care professionals related to patient discharge from hospital. *Informatics for Health and Social Care*, 40(3), pp.198–209. https://doi.org/10.3109/17538157.2013.879150. PMID: 24475936.

Zayas-Cabán, T. (2012). Health information management in the home: A human factors assessment. *Work*, 41(3), pp.315–328.

Chapter 7

Information Management in Nursing Leaders' Operational Decision-Making

Laura-Maria Peltonen

Contents

Introduction

Digitalisation and technological progression has enabled the development and implementation of advanced information and communication technologies to support improved information use in the management of nursing and healthcare organisations. Information management has always had its place in managing and administering healthcare services. Still, the increasing pace and amount of information collected and stored offer a means for better knowledge-driven managerial decision-making, a prerequisite for

DOI: 10.4324/9781003054849-7

efficient organisational processes and high-quality healthcare services. From the managerial perspective, data is needed for monitoring, predicting, planning and control. To achieve this, data needs to be selected, pre-processed, altered, mined and interpreted. Consequently, information and communication technologies have become integral tools for healthcare leaders.

Healthcare organisations typically have a hierarchical design with multidisciplinary leadership (Andersson et al., 2003; Lundgrén-Laine et al., 2011). The managerial decision-making of healthcare organisations can be described through strategic, tactical and operational levels (Winter et al., 2001). In addition, decision-making occurs on the clinical level, which refers to care provided to individuals, families and communities. Strategic decisions include long-term goals, tactical decisions are associated with the execution of strategic plans and operational decisions are about executing the day-to-day activities in an organisation or a unit. Much information is produced, processed and stored regarding service users, care and delivery every day. Information management focuses typically on patients, the workforce and materials. This information is managed in the organisation horizontally and vertically to meet the differing demands of actors on these levels (Murtola et al., 2013; Nyssen, 2007). A simplified illustration of information management for healthcare leaders on different decision-making levels in the organisation is presented in Figure 7.1.

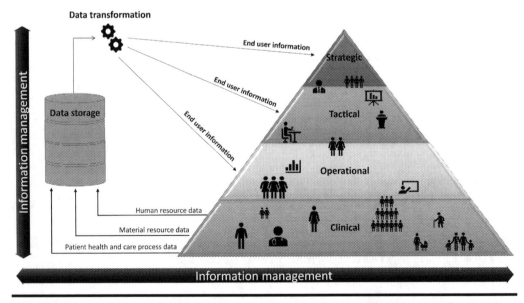

Figure 7.1   Information management for leaders on different decision-making levels in healthcare organisations (modified from Murtola et al., 2013).

Operations management can be defined as managing resources to produce and deliver products or services (Slack et al., 2010), such as healthcare services. Operations management in care delivery is a complex and demanding task due to numerous professionals and specialities, unexpected and sometimes persistent changing situations, constant interruptions and a vast amount of scattered information. There is ample research on operations management in organisation and management science. However, the operations management of health service delivery is much less explored, particularly from the perspective of how information supports decision-making when overseeing a specific unit during a particular shift.

In general, the managerial process includes several tasks, such as coordination (McCallin & Frankson, 2010; Weiss & Tappen, 2015), planning, organisation, command and control (Marquis & Huston, 2017; McCallin & Frankson, 2010; Weiss & Tappen, 2015). The management of a unit is a process that constitutes directing through the arrangement and use of available resources, typically discerned from the leadership function, which focuses on influencing behaviours of the people within the organisation (Marquis & Huston, 2017; Weiss & Tappen, 2015). Unit leaders are responsible for the operations management; however, outside of office hours, the responsibility for acute managerial tasks is typically delegated to chosen staff members who are on-site during a particular shift. Information needs of these actors differ by role and time of day (Peltonen et al., 2019). Consequently, information technology needs to be flexible to address user-specific needs.

Decisions made by nursing leaders have a broad-reaching influence on care delivery, as nursing leaders are responsible for the largest professional group in the healthcare setting. Nurse leaders have typically relied on information technologies for workforce planning and deployment tools in the longer-term operations management (Burton et al., 2018; Griffiths et al., 2020). But far less technologies have been developed for nursing leaders' ad hoc-decision-making.

Although research on the impact of information in operations management of health service delivery is scarce, there is evidence to show that poorly coordinated human and material resources decrease the quality of care and employee satisfaction (Johansson et al., 2016; Kane et al., 2007; Raup, 2008). Inadequate personnel resources increase patient mortality (Aiken et al., 2014; Junttila et al., 2016; Kane et al., 2007; Needleman et al., 2011), and reduce coping with work (Cummings et al., 2010). Further, research has shown that operational leaders' decision-making is associated with staff performance, outcomes and intention to stay, as well as patient safety (Agnew & Flin, 2014; Cummings et al., 2010), satisfaction and health outcomes (Cummings et al., 2010; Gunawan & Aungsuroch, 2017), implementation of research evidence (Gifford et al., 2007) and effectiveness of care (Cummings et al., 2010). This chapter focuses on the operational decision-making of healthcare services with an emphasis on information management and tools available to nursing leaders.

Managerial Decision-making and the Role of Data and Information in Care Delivery

Researchers from many disciplines have been interested in studying how decisions are made and what factors are connected to the decision-making process and the decisions made. Numerous theories and models have been developed to describe the decision-making of individuals in different environments and situations. In nursing, the approach is often analytical or intuitive (Cader et al. 2005; Lauri et al., 2001; Lauri & Salanterä, 1998). The analytical decision is a systematic traceable process, which is based on the best obtainable data, information and knowledge. It is seen as a more reliable and transparent approach to managerial decision-making than the intuitive decision, which is based on knowledge and experience of the decision-maker without a systematic process that later could be described and replicated (Saaty, 2008). The analytical decision process is largely dependent upon access to relevant, measurable and scalable data.

Prior research has shown that individuals' personal characteristics, such as gender, experience, preferences, values and ways of thinking, influence the decision made (Marquis & Huston, 2017) and the chosen decision-making model (Lauri et al., 2001). Although there is individual and situational-related divergence in how individuals make decisions, less experienced leaders usually follow linear decision-making processes, while senior individuals also use the experience to be more effective when making decisions (Asamani et al., 2013, McCallin & Frankson, 2010). Research has also indicated that nursing professionals resort to intuitive decision-making rather than analytical decision-making when rapid decision-making is vital (Lauri et al., 2001; Lauri & Salanterä, 1998). Many decision-making models describe decision-making as a process, which constitutes several steps. While the number of steps varies between models, they typically include the following:

1. Defining the problem
2. Seeking information needed
3. Determining alternatives for a solution
4. Deciding the best alternative to follow
5. Evaluating the decision made

Operational leaders' decision-making processes and related factors are described in Figure 7.2.

The content of decisions made by nursing leaders in operations management include the organisation of resources and work regarding staff, materials and patient care (Andersson et al., 2003; Asamani et al., 2013; Lundgrén-Laine et al., 2011; McCallin & Frankson, 2010; Siirala et al., 2016) as well as issues related to education, counselling, administration, patient safety and quality of care (Admi & Eilon-Moshe, 2016; Asamani et al., 2013; McCallin & Frankson, 2010). Supporting nursing leaders with appropriate information technology to obtain necessary and flawless information at the right time supports optimal decisions.

Data and information play pivotal functions in operations management. Accurate and timely data and information are key for achieving situational awareness, which means that the leader recognises relevant elements in the setting at a specific point in time, comprehends the meaning of these elements and is able to project the situation for the near future (Endsley, 1995).

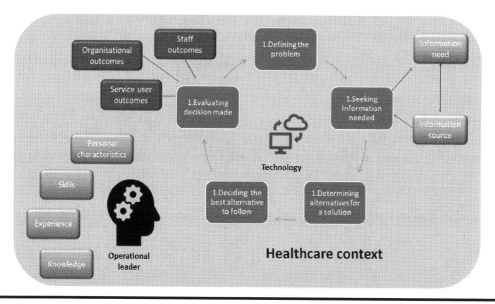

Figure 7.2   Operational leaders' decision-making and related factors.

Situational awareness is currently receiving an increasing amount of attention in healthcare, particularly from an operations management perspective (Kontio et al., 2013; Lundgrén-Laine et al., 2013; Norri-Sederholm et al., 2015). Lack of situational awareness presents a serious risk to patient safety, staff work and well-being and quality of care delivered. Therefore, it is crucial that leaders devote attention to the substance, accuracy, timeliness, format and accessibility of data and information needed at the point of decision-making.

Situational awareness can be enhanced through numerous information management solutions for capturing, storing, processing and distributing data for different purposes in healthcare. These solutions are sensitive to data and information that are being produced and collected at an increasing pace. Big data is generally considered an organisational asset. Big data enables the creation of actionable ideas to monitor, support and improve the organisational processes (Russom, 2011). Various techniques are available for analysing these large amounts of data within the data analytics process. The data analytics process is often divided into phases including assessment, selection, cleaning, filtering, visualisation, analysis, interpretation and assessment of results (Runkler, 2016). Innovations for selecting and analysing real-time data may help predict patterns and create knowledge for forecasting future outcomes as means to improve healthcare quality (Sensmeier, 2016). However, the source data must be accurate and valid, complete and up-to-date and measurable and scalable for purposeful and reliable use (Zygiaris, 2018). Selecting the content and describing the requirements for the expected outcome based on available and needed data and information for operations management is the first step in improving information management and developing tools to better support nursing leaders' work in operations management.

Since fragmented data does not support a more holistic view, nursing leaders have traditionally integrated and processed patient and staffing related information through a data warehouse approach. Data is stored in a structured way based on a pre-defined schema (Junttila et al., 2007). This approach is limited to a fixed configuration and may not support innovation later when analysing the data unless particular attention is given to ensuring scalable and measurable data are collected. While this approach is maturing so that ad hoc-decisions can be addressed, nursing leaders need real-time operations management based on real-time access to data and information. Currently, some healthcare organisations are adopting a data lake approach, where data is stored in its raw format. This may be in a structured (i.e., takes a pre-defined format or model), a semi-structured (i.e., takes some degree of format but is not fully organised) or an unstructured (i.e., lacks pre-defined format) form. This enables far more analytical possibilities and hindsight when analysing data and developing information management from a nursing leader's perspective. At this time, this approach usually requires custom-made user interfaces for nursing leaders so that they can access and use the data.

While data analytics can enhance the efficiency of operations management through predictive models and real-time analytics, this support depends on the level of organisational maturity to ensure that big data is available (Sousa et al., 2019). Well-designed information systems architectures that support data and information management in healthcare organisations are needed to support health service delivery appropriately. However, designing optimal information systems is not sufficient alone. Nurse leaders need to be competent in informatics (Strudwick et al., 2019a, b; Collins et al., 2017). They need resources to support them with data management and analytics. An infrastructure that includes informatics specialists with an understanding of nursing is required on all levels in healthcare organisations to ensure appropriate information management in nursing from strategic to operational levels of decision-making. This level of support could be accomplished by establishing nursing science big data centres that share resources, unite language standards, advance nursing databases and create knowledge system constructions (Zhu et al., 2019). Education on and implementation of standardised terminologies and documentation guidelines are primary means to improve the content stored in big data sets. But, to ensure data quality, data collected in these systems also need systematic quality assessment (Junttila et al., 2007).

Information Needs and Sources in Healthcare Operational Decision-making

An information need may be described as an item needed for solving a problem (Timmins, 2006) or by recognising inadequate knowledge to meet an aim at a particular occasion (Ormandy, 2011). Information needs of the professionals responsible for operations management differ by responsibilities and accountabilities. Some information needs are shared regardless of profession, timepoint or unit, such as patient information, staffing and materials (Andersson et al., 2003; Kontio et al., 2013; Lundgrén-Laine et al., 2013;

Norri-Sederholm et al., 2015) while others differ. For example, nurses' information needs cover general staffing, material and patient information, while physicians' information needs typically focus on the patients' medical diagnoses and interventions (Lundgrén-Laine et al., 2013; Peltonen et al., 2019). Hence, nurse leaders need different data for their information systems in operations management when compared to physicians.

Nurse leaders addressing operations management need large amounts of easily obtainable real-time and accurate information to support their decision-making. Their information needs are aligned with their responsibilities. They typically are concerned with care needs and processes, organisation of work, clinical care–related treatments, examinations and procedures, as well as the allocation of material and staffing resources (Peltonen et al., 2018; Lundgrén-Laine et al., 2013; Andersson et al., 2003; Asamani et al., 2013; Lundgrén-Laine et al., 2011; McCallin & Frankson, 2010; Siirala et al., 2016). Earlier research has indicated that information needs may be associated with both the unit's size and the nurse's experience (Lundgrén-Laine et al., 2013). Nonetheless, research exploring ad hoc-decision-making in operations management emphasises a clear need for real-time information about the situation in the organisation or unit (Kontio et al., 2013; Lundgrén-Laine et al., 2013) when compared to decision-making targeting the near-future or beyond. Therefore, the conventional warehouse-based approaches do not support ad hoc-decision-making in the operations management sufficiently.

There are different ways to describe how information is managed in decision-making. One commonly used theory in nursing is the information-processing theory (Lauri & Salanterä, 1998; Thompson et al., 2017), which articulates that decision-making is done based on earlier knowledge, collecting information, generating alternatives, as well as forming and testing hypotheses (Newell, 1989; Newell & Simon, 1972). Aligned with this, the information seeker first identifies an information need, then turns to information sources to obtain information necessary, either succeeds or fails in obtaining information needed and then is satisfied or alternatively continues with the information-seeking behaviour (Wilson, 1981).

Optimal information management, which builds on user-centred and intuitive solutions, best supports operations management of health service delivery. Unfortunately, it is the case that unnecessary time is currently spent on trying to find information not available, out-of-date, or located in dispersed places (Kontio et al., 2013). Information sources include individuals as well as paper-based and digital systems (Andersson et al., 2003; Kontio et al., 2013; Peltonen et al., 2016), which are located within and outside of the unit. Moreover, some information is only found within the leader's mind as knowledge or experience (Peltonen et al., 2016). Healthcare operational leaders have reported serious needs for improved information management tools and solutions to improve speed and access to important information, and a need for more intuitive interfaces that assemble all necessary information into one place for display (Peltonen et al., 2018a, b).

Technologies Available for Nursing Leaders' Operational Decision-making

Healthcare information systems are often divided into clinical and administrative systems. Clinical systems focus directly on patient care, such as the electronic health record or the order entry system. In contrast, administrative systems support care delivery, such as human resource management systems and scheduling systems (Marquis & Huston, 2017; Zytkowski et al., 2018). The administrative systems can further be divided into management information systems and communication systems (Clément, 2015). The systems developed for the healthcare setting can also be divided into three types, including information systems, which collect, store and display data and information; decision support systems, which help to interpret, integrate and understand the information; and expert systems, which are able to give predictions and recommendations to solve particular problems (ANA, 2015).

Digitalisation has enabled the processing and use of vast amounts of data and information to support decision-making on all organisational levels. Most research and developmental work have so far mainly focused on clinical management and the development of tools to support this. A much smaller portion of work has targeted the development or evaluation of the impact of tools to support healthcare leaders' information management and decision-making, particularly from the operational leaders' ad hoc-decision-making perspective (Murtola et al., 2013). One common characteristic of systems available for healthcare leaders is that they typically only serve one purpose at a time, such as scheduling, patient classification, workload management, (Choi et al., 2014; Clément, 2015; Kerfoot & Smith, 2015; Rauhala & Fagerström 2004), patient care management (Choi et al., 2014), cost accounting (Choi et al., 2014; Clément, 2015), human resource management (Clément, 2015; Pulido et al., 2014), material resource management, fiscal resources (Clément, 2015), as well as quality surveillance and quality improvement (Clément, 2015; Jeffs et al., 2014; Kinnunen-Luovi et al., 2014). Based on a previous review of the literature, scheduling programmes, nursing cost-related programmes and patient care management programmes may effectively save time and support nursing care. However, there is a lack of quality in the evidence (Choi et al., 2014). Nonetheless, operational leaders currently use several information systems simultaneously to collect important information for their decision-making (Peltonen et al., 2018a, b), which makes information management far less effective.

Information systems, which integrate information into an overall view of an organisation's or unit's situation for healthcare leaders, are slowly emerging (Jeffs et al., 2014; Krugman & Sanders, 2016). However, most systems still provide the information retrospectively without real-time information support. Further, more comprehensive systems that integrate the information for operations management are still lacking (Yoo et al., 2016). With the advancement of technologies such as predictive algorithms and natural language processing, there is enormous potential in supporting nursing leaders' operations management and developing expert systems for ad hoc-decision-making. Given that many advanced technologies are still in the technology development phase, there is still a long way to go before safe adoption into the clinical setting.

Implications for Practice and Research

Information systems are associated with improved efficiency, higher quality of care and better productivity, as well as lower costs. However, healthcare operations management is to date poorly supported by information technology (Peltonen et al., 2018a, b), and research on the impact of managerial information systems on the patient, staffing and organisational outcomes is scarce. Knowledge-driven healthcare operations management needs the implementation of user-centred and intuitive information systems, which provide timely, accurate and important information tailored to the specific user needs and displays it in an easily interpretable format. In addition to paying attention to standards and semantic interoperability, developing such systems requires the involvement of end-users throughout the technology development process to ensure appropriateness and feasibility. However, research shows that nurses are still seldomly involved in these processes (Hyyppönen et al., 2018). Increasing nursing leaders' engagement in all phases of the technology development process and healthcare organisations' information management and systems architecture planning will support more appropriate advancement of health service delivery. Future work needs to focus on developing, implementing and evaluating advanced, intuitive, flexible and effective systems that better support nursing leaders in operational management and ad hoc-decision-making in particular. Optimal information management supports optimal decision-making, supporting good leadership and improving organisational, service user and staffing outcomes.

It is important to keep in mind that there are always risks to be acknowledged when adopting new technologies in the healthcare setting. Safe use of technology is the responsibility of the vendor, the organisation and the professional using it. This emphasises the need for a systematic plan on ensuring competencies of the producers of data and the users of implemented technologies within an organisation. For example, regarding artificial intelligence-based technologies, nursing leaders need to understand issues with explainability, user knowledge and skills requirements, risks with biased algorithms and data security aspects (Ronquillo et al., 2021). Hence, future work is needed from the operational leaders' point of view on how to ensure competence when using constantly renewable technologies from various organisational perspectives with an emphasis on understanding the technology content and functionality.

Conclusions

Nursing leaders' operations management is not sufficiently supported by accessible technologies in healthcare organisations. Information needs vary based on a broad spectrum of responsibilities and related decisions concerning the organisation of resources and work regarding staff, materials and patient care. Decisions made based on inaccurate information may decrease healthcare performance. Currently, information systems available to nursing leaders mainly exist to serve a single purpose at a time and they rarely provide a holistic, instantaneous and real-time view of the situation. While the information for solving managerial issues in operations management is somewhat available, information for ad hoc-decision-making in operations management is scattered and not available in real-time. For optimal decision-making, nursing leaders need improved tools that provide real-time knowledge-based comprehensive views of their unit and organisation in one and the same display and configured based on each user's specific needs. Supporting decision-making with appropriate tools would bring about improved service user, staffing and organisational outcomes.

Another approach to improve nursing leaders' information management includes taking better advantage of big data. This has the potential to provide nursing leaders with better information for knowledge-driven operational decision-making. Nonetheless, it is important to acknowledge the weakness of the data used as there may be inaccuracies in the input data that do not reflect reality. This emphasises the need for appropriate use of standard terminologies and systematic quality checks to ensure the quality of data collected and stored. However, sufficient technological maturity in the organisation is needed, with appropriate competencies, informatics-related infrastructure, roles and technologies to support nursing leaders' use of big data. Nursing leaders also need to have sufficient competence in informatics themselves to describe and communicate their needs and requirements regarding information desired and tools needed to support their access to important information. Nursing leaders are the only ones who can pinpoint what they need. Their active engagement in developing information management architectures and tools to better support their needs is therefore crucial.

Nursing is evolving rapidly, which influences roles, tasks and requirements for nurses and nursing leaders. Future projections on anticipated changes in nursing show a shift towards increased adoption of technologies such as virtual reality and the Internet of Things to support care delivery; digital health and virtual models of care; an increased use of data analytics, artificial intelligence and system automation; new roles for nurses as system navigators; and an increased need for informatics prepared nurses (Buchanan et al., 2020; Booth et al., 2021). Further, the adoption of new technologies has the potential to improve service user, staff and organisational outcomes. Combined with the evolving roles in nursing and change in care delivery, this increases the expectations for nursing leaders, who need to prepare themselves with a vision for the future and necessary competencies for leading this change. Appropriate strategic planning and tactical implementation of information and communication technologies to meet future demands will aid to achieve the quadruple aim to optimise health system performance (Bodenheimer & Sinskey, 2014).

References

Admi, H., & Eilon-Moshe, Y. (2016). Do hospital shift charge nurses from different cultures experience similar stress? An international cross sectional study. *International Journal of Nursing Studies*, 63, pp.48–57.

Agnew, C., & Flin, R. (2014). Senior charge nurses' leadership behaviours in relation to hospital ward safety: A mixed method study. *International Journal of Nursing Studies*, 51(5), pp.768–780.

Aiken, L. H., Sloane, D. M., Bruyneel, L., Van den Heede, K., Griffiths, P., Busse, R., Diomidous, M., Kinnunen, J., Kózka, M., Lesaffre, E., & McHugh, M. D. (2014). Nurse staffing and education and hospital mortality in nine European countries: A retrospective observational study. *The Lancet*, 383(9931), pp.1824–1830. https://doi.org/10.1016/S0140-6736(13)62631-8

ANA (American Nurses Association). (2015). Nursing informatics: Scope and standards of practice. Silver Spring, MD: American Nurses Publishing.

Andersson, A., Hallberg, N., & Timpka, T. (2003). A model for interpreting work and information management in process-oriented healthcare organisations. *International Journal of Medical Informatics*, 72(1–3), pp.47–56.

Asamani, J. A., Kwafo, E. O., & Ansah-Ofei, A. M. (2013). Planning among nurse managers in district hospitals in Ghana. *Nursing Management*, 20(8), pp.26–31.

Bodenheimer, T., & Sinsky, C. (2014). From triple to quadruple aim: Care of the patient requires care of the provider. *The Annals of Family Medicine*, 12(6), pp.573–576.

Booth, R., Strudwick, G., McMurray, J., Chan, R., Cotton, K., & Cooke, S. (2021). The future of *nursing* informatics in a digitally-enabled world. In *Introduction to nursing informatics*. Cham: Springer, pp.395–417.

Buchanan, C., Howitt, M. L., Wilson, R., Booth, R. G., Risling, T., & Bamford, M. (2020). Predicted influences of artificial intelligence on the domains of nursing: Scoping review. *JMIR Nursing*, 3(1), p.e23939.

Burton, C., Rycroft-Malone, J., Williams, L., Davies, S., McBride, A., Hall, B., Rowlands, A. M., Jones, A., Fisher, D., Jones, M., & Caulfield, M. (2018). NHS managers' use of nursing workforce planning and deployment technologies: A realist synthesis. *Health Services and Delivery Research*, 6(36).

Cader, R., Campbell, S., & Watson, D. (2005). Cognitive continuum theory in nursing decision-making. *Journal of Advanced Nursing*, 49(4), pp.397–405. https://doi.org/10.1111/j.1365-2648.2004.03303.x

Choi, M., Yang, Y. L., & Lee S. M. (2014). Effectiveness of nursing management information systems: A systematic review. *Healthcare Informatics Research*, 20(4), 249–257.

Clément, H. (2015). Administration applications. In K. J. Hannah, P. Hussey, M. A. Kennedy, & M. J. Ball, eds., *Introduction to nursing informatics*. 4th ed. London: Springer, pp.215–230.

Collins, S., Yen, P. Y., Phillips, A., & Kennedy, M. K. (2017). Nursing informatics competency assessment for the nurse leader: The Delphi study. *Journal of Nursing Administration*, 47(4), pp.212–218. https://doi.org/10.1097/NNA.0000000000000467

Cummings, G. G., MacGregor, T., Davey, M., Lee, H., Wong, C. A., Lo, E., Muise, M., & Stafford, E. (2010). Leadership styles and outcome patterns for the nursing workforce and work environment: A systematic review. *International Journal of Nursing Studies*, 47(3), pp.363–385.

Endsley, M. R. (1995). Toward a theory of situation awareness in dynamic systems. *Human Factors*, 37(1), pp. 32–64. https://doi.org/10.1518/001872095779049543

Gifford, W., Davies, B., Edunits, N., Griffin, P., & Lybanon, V. (2007). Managerial leadership for nurses' use of research evidence: An integrative review of the literature. *Worldviews on Evidence Based Nursing*, 4(3), pp.126–145.

Griffiths, P., Saville, C., Ball, J., Jones, J., Pattison, N., Monks, T., & the Safer Nursing Care Study Group. (2020). Nursing workload, nurse staffing methodologies and tools: A systematic scoping review and discussion. *International Journal of Nursing Studies*, 103, pp.103487. https://doi.org/10.1016/j.ijnurstu.2019.103487

Gunawan, J., & Aungsuroch, Y. (2017). Managerial competence of first-line nurse managers: A concept analysis. *International Journal of Nursing Practice*, 23(1), pp.1–7. https://doi.org/10.1111/ijn.12502

Hyppönen, H., Lääveri, T., Hahtela, N., Suutarla, A., Sillanpää, K., Kinnunen, U. M., Ahonen, O., Rajalahti, E., Kaipio, J., Heponiemi, T., & Saranto, K. (2018). Kyvykkäille käyttäjille fiksut järjestelmät? Sairaanhoitajien arviot potilastieto-järjestelmistä 2017, *Finnish Journal of eHealth and eWelfare (FinJeHeW)*, 10(1). https://doi.org/10.23996/fjhw.65363

Jeffs L., Beswick S., Lo J., Lai Y., Chhun A., & Campbell H. (2014). Insights from staff nurses and managers on unit–specific nursing performance dashboards: A qualitative study. *BMJ Quality & Safety*, 23(12), pp.1001–1006.

Johansson, G., Andersson, L., Gustafsson, B., & Sandahl, C. (2016). Between being and doing – the nature of *leadership* of first–line nurse managers and registered nurses. *Journal of Clinical Nursing*, 19(17–18), pp.2619–2628.

Junttila, K., Meretoja, R., Seppälä, A., Tolppanen, E. M., Ala-Nikkola, T., & Silvennoinen, L. (2007). Data *warehouse* approach to nursing management. *Journal of Nursing Management*, 15(2), pp.155–161. https://doi.org/10.1111/j.1365-2834.2007.00690.x

Junttila, J. K., Koivu, A., Fagerström, L., Haatainen, K., & Nykänen, P. (2016). Hospital mortality and optimality of nursing workload: A study on the predictive validity of the RAFAELA nursing *intensity* and staffing system. *International Journal of Nursing Studies*, 60, pp.46–53. https://doi.org/10.1016/j.ijnurstu.2016.03.008

Kane, R. L., Shamliyan, T. A., Mueller, C., Duval, S., & Wilt, T. J. (2007). The association of registered nurse staffing *levels* and patient outcomes: Systematic review and meta-analysis. *Medical Care*, 45(12), pp.1195–1204.

Kerfoot, K. M., & Smith, K. (2015). Nurse scheduling and credentialing systems, In V. K. Saba, & K. A. McCormick, eds., *Essentials of nursing informatics*. 6th ed. New York: McGrawHill, pp.323–331.

Kinnunen–Luovi, K., Saarnio, R., & Isola, A. (2014). Safety incidents involving confused and forgetful older patients in a specialised care setting: Analysis of the safety incidents reported to the HaiPro *reporting* system. *Journal of Clinical Nursing*, 23(17–18), pp.2442–2450.

Kontio, E., Lundgrén-Laine, H., Kontio, J., Korvenranta, H., & Salanterä, S. (2013). Information *utilization* in tactical decision making of middle management health managers. *Computers Informatics Nursing*, 31(1), pp.9–16. https://doi.org/10.1097/NXN.0b013e318261f192

Krugman, M. E., & Sanders, C. L. (2016). Implementing a nurse manager pro-file to improve unit *performance. Journal of Nursing Administration*, 46(6), pp.345–351.

Lauri, S., & Salanterä, S. (1998). Decision-making models in different fields of nurs-ing. *Research in Nursing & Health*, 21(5), pp.443–452.

Lauri, S., Salanterä, S., Chalmers, K., Ekman, S. L., Kim, H. S., Käppeli, S., & MacLeod, M. (2001). An *exploratory* study of clinical decision-making in five countries. *Journal of Nursing Scholarship*, 33(1), pp.83–90.

Lundgrén-Laine, H., Kontio, E., Perttilä, J., Korvenranta, H., Forsström, J., & Salanterä, S. (2011). Managing daily intensive care activities: An observational study concerning ad hoc decision making of charge nurses and intensivists. *Critical Care*, 15(4), pp.1–10.

Lundgrén-Laine, H., Kontio, E., Kauko, T., Korvenranta, H., Forsström, J., & Salanterä, S. (2013). *National* survey focusing on the crucial information needs of intensive care charge nurses and intensivists: Same goal, different demands. *BMC Medical Informatics and Decision Making* 13, p.15. https://doi.org/10.11 86/1472-6947-13-15

Marquis, B. L., & Huston, C. J. (2017). *Leadership roles and management functions in nursing: Theory and application*. 9th ed. St. Louis: Lippincott Williams & Wilkins Inc.

McCallin, A. M., & Frankson, C. (2010). The role of the charge nurse manager: A descriptive exploratory study. *Journal of Nursing Management*, 18(3), pp.319–325.

Murtola, LM., Lundgrén-Laine, H., & Salanterä, S. (2013). Information sys-tems in hospitals: A review article from a nursing management perspec-tive. *International Journal of Networking and Virtual Organisations*, 13(1), pp.81–100.

Needleman, J., Buerhaus, P., Pankratz, V. S., Leibson, C. L., Stevens, S. R., & Harris, M. (2011). Nurse staffing and inpatient hospital mortality. *New England Journal of Medicine*, 364(11), pp.1037–1045. https://doi.org/10.1056/NEJMsa1001025

Newell, A. (1989). Putting it all together. In D. Klahr, & K. Kotovsky, eds., *Complex information processing*. Mahwah, NJ: Erlbaum, pp.399–440.

Newell, A., & Simon, H. A. (1972). *Human problem solving*, 104(9). Englewood Cliffs, NJ: Prentice-Hall.

Norri-Sederholm, T., Paakkonen, H., Kurola, J., & Saranto, K. (2015). Situational awareness and information flow in prehospital emergency medical care from the perspective of paramedic field supervisors: A scenario–based study. *Scandinavian Journal of Trauma, Resuscitation and Emergency Medicine* 23(4), pp.1–9.

Nyssen, A. S. (2007). Coordination in hospitals: Organized or emergent process? *Cognition, Technology & Work*, 9(3), pp.149–154.

Ormandy, P. (2011). Defining information need in health–assimilating complex the-ories derived from information science. *Health Expectations*, 14(1), pp.92–104.

Peltonen, L. M., Lundgrén-Laine, H., & Salanterä, S. (2016). Information manage-ment in the daily care coordination in the intensive care unit. In H. Li, P. Nykänen, R. Suomi, N. Wickramasinghe, C. Widén, M. Zhan et al., eds.,

Communications in computer and information science 636: Building sustainable health ecosystems. Berlin: Springer, pp.1–15. https://doi.org/10.1007/978-3-319-44672-1_19

Peltonen, L. M., Junttila, K., & Salanterä, S. (2018a). Front-Line Physicians' Satisfaction with Information Systems in Hospitals. In A. Ugon et al., eds., *Building Continents of Knowledge in Oceans of Data: The Future of Co-Created eHealth Proceedings of MIE2018.* IOS Press, pp.865–869.

Peltonen, L. M., Junttila, K., & Salanterä, S. (2018b). Nursing leaders' satisfaction with information systems in the day-to-day operations management in hospital units. In A. K. Rotegård et al., eds., *Nursing informatics 2018.* IOS Press, pp.203–207.

Peltonen, L. M., Lundgrén-Laine, H., Siirala, E., Löyttyniemi, E., Aantaa, R., & Salanterä, S. (2018c). Assessing managerial information needs: Modification and evaluation of the hospital shift Leaders' information needs questionnaire. *Journal of Nursing Management,* 26(2), pp.108–119. https://doi.org/10.1111/jonm.12515

Peltonen, L. M., Siirala, E., Junttila, K., Lundgrén-Laine, H., Vahlberg, T., Löyttyniemi, E., Aantaa, R., & Salanterä, S. (2019). Information needs in day-to-day operations management in hospital units: A cross-sectional national survey. *Journal of Nursing Management,* 27(2), pp.233–244.

Pulido, R., Aguirre, A. M., Ortega–Mier, M., García–Sánchez, Á., & Méndez, C. A. (2014). Managing daily surgery schedules in a teaching hospital: A mixed–integer optimization approach. *BMC Health Services Research,* 14(1), pp.1–13.

Rauhala, A., & Fagerström, L. (2004). Determining optimal nursing intensity: The RAFAELA method. *Journal of Advanced Nursing,* 45(4), pp.351–359.

Raup, G. H. (2008). The impact of ED nurse manager leadership style on staff nurse turnover and *patient* satisfaction in academic health center hospitals. *Journal of Emergency Nursing,* 34(5), pp.403–409.

Ronquillo, C. E., Peltonen, L. M., Pruinelli, L., Chu, C. H., Bakken, S., Beduschi, A., Cato, K., Hardiker, N., Junger, A., Michalowski, M., & Nyrup, R. (2021). Artificial intelligence in nursing: Priorities and opportunities from an international invitational think-tank of the nursing and artificial intelligence leadership collaborative. *Journal of Advanced Nursing,* 77(9), pp.3707–3717. https://doi.org/10.1111/jan.14855

Runkler, T. A. (2016). *Data analytics.* New York: Springer Fachmedien Wiesbaden. https://doi.org/10.1007/978-3-658-14075-5_1

Russom, P. (2011). Big data analytics. TDWI best practices report. *Fourth Quarter,* 19(4), pp.1–34.

Saaty, T. L. (2008). Decision making with the analytic hierarchy process. *International Journal of Services Sciences,* 1(1), pp.83–98.

Sensmeier, J. (2016). Understanding the impact of big data on nursing knowledge. *Nursing Critical Care,* 11(2), pp.11–13.

Siirala, E., Peltonen, L. M., Lundgrén-Laine, H., Salanterä, S., & Junttila, K. (2016). Nurse managers' decision-making in daily unit operation in peri-operative settings: A cross-sectional descriptive study. *Journal of Nursing Management,* 24(6), pp.806–815. https://doi.org/10.1111/jonm.12385

Slack, N., Chambers, S., & Johnston, R. (2010). *Operations management.* 6th ed. London: Pearson education.

Sousa, M. J., Pesqueira, A. M., Lemos, C., Sousa, M., & Rocha, Á. (2019). Decision-making based on big data analytics for people management in healthcare organizations. *Journal of Medical Systems*, 43(9), pp.1–10.

Strudwick, G., Nagle, L., Kassam, I., Pahwa, M., & Sequeira, L. (2019a). Informatics competencies for nurse leaders: A scoping review. *Journal of Nursing Administration.* 49(6), pp.323–330. https://doi.org/10.1097/NNA.0000000000000760

Strudwick, G., Nagle, L. M., Morgan, A., Kennedy, M. A., Currie, L. M., Lo, B., & White, P. (2019b). Adapting and validating informatics competencies for senior nurse leaders in the Canadian context: Results of a Delphi study. *International Journal of Medical Informatics*, 129, pp.211–218. https://doi.org/10.1016/j.ijmedinf.2019.06.012

Thompson, S., Moorley, C., & Barratt, J. (2017). A comparative study on the clinical decision–making processes of nurse practitioners vs. medical doctors using scenarios in a secondary care environment. *Journal of Advanced Nursing*, 73(5), pp.1097–1110.

Timmins, F. (2006). Exploring the concept of 'information need'. *International Journal of Nursing Practice*, 12(6), pp.375–381.

Weiss, S. A., & Tappen, R. M. (2015). *Essentials of nursing leadership and management.* 6th ed. Philadelphia, PA: Davis Company.

Wilson, T. D. (1981). On user studies and information needs. *Journal of Documentation*, 37(1), pp.3–15.

Winter, A. F., Ammenwerth, E., Bott, O. J., Brigl, B., Buchauer, A., Gräber, S., Grant, A., Häber, A., Hasselbring, W., Haux, R., Heinrich, A., Janssen, H., Kock, I., Penger, O. S., Prokosch, H. U., Terstappen, A., & Winter, A.(2001). Strategic information management plans: The basis for systematic information management in hospitals. *International Journal of Medical Informatics*, 64(2–3), pp.99–109.

Yoo, S., Hwang, H., & Jheon, S. (2016). Hospital information systems: Experience at the fully digitized Seoul National University Bundang Hospital. *Journal of Thoracic Disease*, 8(Suppl 8), pp.S637–641.

Zhu, R., Han, S., Su, Y., Zhang, C., Yu, Q., & Duan, Z. (2019). The application of big data and the development of nursing science: A discussion paper. *International Journal of Nursing Sciences*, 6(2), pp.229–234.

Zygiaris, S. (2018). *Database management systems: A business-oriented approach using ORACLE, MySQL and MS access.* Emerald Group Publishing.

Zytkowski, M., Paschke, S., Mastrian, K., & McGonigle, D. (2018). Administrative information systems. In D. McGonigle, & K. G. Mastrian, eds., *Nursing informatics and the foundation of knowledge.* 4th ed. Burlington: Jones & Barlett Learning, pp.189–206.

Chapter 8

Informatics in Large Health Systems: Organization, Transformation and Nursing Informatics Leadership Perspectives

Sheila Ochylski and Rebecca Freeman

Contents

DOI: 10.4324/9781003054849-8

Introduction

A Brief History of Nursing Informatics

The U.S. Department of Veterans Affairs

The U.S. Department of Veterans Affairs (VA) has one of the largest nursing staff of any healthcare system in the world. Numbering over 116,000 nationwide, the VA integrated nursing team, composed of Registered Nurses (RNs), advanced practice Registered Nurses (APRNs), Licensed Practical/Vocational Nurses (LPNs/LVNs) and nursing assistants, provides comprehensive, complex and compassionate care to the nation's Veterans to maintain health throughout the care continuum.

Within VA, nurse informaticists have a long legacy of innovation to define and use data to build knowledge within the nursing domain (Deckro et al., 2021). The legacy began in the 1970s with the innovative efforts to create the Computerized Patient Record System (CPRS) and again in the 1990s with the development of the Bar Code Medication Administration (BCMA) application. This program has become the hallmark for current medication administration records (Brown et al., 2003). In the 1990s, CPRS was released, and clinical application coordinator (CAC) roles emerged within nursing informatics to support it as client-server programming within a graphical user interface (GUI). Nursing informaticists in the Veterans Health Administration (VHA), the healthcare division within VA, have been instrumental in improving, supporting and informing both CPRS, clinical information systems and BCMA across the VHA system development life cycle. Nursing informaticists within VHA continue to evolve and build upon these foundational nursing informatics strategies to seek opportunities to provide excellence in patient care to our nation's Veterans and their families. Today in VHA, there are over 500 nurses with an informatics specialty who have graduated from university-based training programs are certified in the specialty of nursing informatics.

Non-VA Large Health Systems

Many of us may have seen a copy of Florence Nightingale's 1858 'coxcomb' pie chart (Figure 8.1), detailing the causes of mortality in the Army of the East in the Crimean War.

Nightingale was an early statistician and perhaps the first nurse informaticist—a trailblazer not just for nursing, but for a methodical, data-driven approach to analysis and care. Academic literature referred to nursing

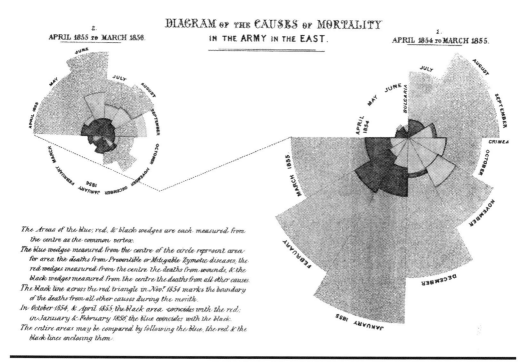

Figure 8.1   Percentage of organizations undertaking different types of change (Gartner Inc., 2017).

and computers in the 1960s. The first conference on nursing and computers was held in the 1970s in the United States, and in 1988 the first graduate program in nursing informatics was established in the United States at the University of Maryland (Cummins et al., 2016; Ozbolt & Saba, 2008). Nursing informatics was designated a specialty of nursing by the American Nurses Association (ANA) in 1992, with written scope and standards for practice appearing in the years 1994–1995 (ANA, 2014). The recognition of the importance of informatics education and informaticists has continued to evolve. The recent American Association of Colleges of Nursing (AACN) Essentials' Domain 8, finalized in 2021, introduces a new and evolved set of competencies supporting the edict that it is essential that nurses at all levels understand their role and the value of their input in health information technology analysis, planning, implementation and evaluation (AACN, 2021).

Informatics knowledge should be a key part of current state nursing practice. The Office of the National Coordinator for Health IT (ONC) reported that by 2017, 99% of large hospitals possessed certified health record technology (ONC, 2017). Based on conversations with informaticists over the years, the authors have come to believe there are no unique problems in the informatics and implementation space; the trends and challenges are consistent and predictable in most large healthcare systems, regardless of the technology (e.g., EHR, event management, telephony, nurse call, etc.), vendor or time since implementation. The authors will use the remainder of this chapter to discuss those trends with an overarching theme: *the technology itself is less important than the environment in which it is being implemented.*

In terms of the nursing informatics workforce, the Health Information and Management Systems Society (HIMSS) 2020 informatics workforce survey had more than 1,300 respondents and provides an excellent, comprehensive look at the contemporary nursing informatics landscape (HIMSS, 2020). For more than a century, the groundwork laid by Nightingale, the evolution of innovative informatics teams like those in VA and the national/international rise of a strong nursing informatics workforce have evolved the informatics domain itself. However, in the operational side of healthcare, the authors frequently encounter low data literacy and an immature application of informatics from the staff closest to the patient through the executive suite. It is often the case that legacy information technology systems have evolved, but the underlying governance and organizational structures that support and provide education for those systems have not.

The discernment of this situation includes observations of the large health systems landscape. While the world of care providers has become more technologically complex, it often seems as if organizations have lagged to evolve their organizational structures to match the technical advances of systems, applications and devices. A specific focus on the varying job descriptions, duties and impact of evolving healthcare delivery, system and reimbursement models on the role of nurse informaticists follows.

Nursing Informatics: Authors' Observations

The authors have the benefit of years of experience with health IT implementations in various arenas. Four key issues have been identified as key barriers to exemplary informatics leadership in successful health IT implementations: workforce inconsistencies, organizational readiness, education and competency gaps and change management (Jones, 2018). Notice that the key issues with implementing technology and optimizing informatics in large health systems seem to have very little to do with technology.

Workforce Inconsistencies

The title 'informaticist' is not unique to nursing. Physicians traditionally have been designated as medical informaticists and interdisciplinary partners in radiology, lab and pharmacy have had informatics team members for years. The job market shows a variety of informatics positions, which may or may not include nurses. A recent search of the HIMSS Job Mine found informaticist titles for nursing, public health, dental medicine, ambulatory care, and a variety of 'health' and 'clinical' informaticist jobs that were multidisciplinary in nature (HIMSS, 2021). The latest HIMSS nursing informatics workforce survey found nurse informaticists housed in eight different areas of the organization, working under nine different job titles with seven distinct key responsibilities and eight named reporting structures. Respondents collectively identified conflicting IT priorities and organizational structure as their top two barriers to success (HIMSS, 2021). In our experience, these inconsistencies and barriers exist from the bedside (e.g., Super User programs) to the executive suite. An additional barrier of the effective integration of informaticists and practice is the frequent absence of informatics competencies in the novice-to-expert (Benner, 1984) development pathway of nurse residencies, orientation and preceptorship, clinical ladder opportunities and position descriptions, even in large healthcare systems.

The Chief Nursing Informatics Officer (CNIO) is often tasked with leading this transformation and integration of informatics. Jackson and Ross (2019) discussed the evolving role of the CNIO as one to support the interdisciplinary informatics team to health IT transformation and the innovative utilization of data while Murphy (2011) described the evolving role of the CNIO as generally a senior informatics nurse guiding implementations and optimizing health information technology (HIT) (Jackson & Ross, 2019; Murphy, 2011). There is still room for growth; the 2020 HIMSS Workforce Survey found that only 41% of nurse informaticists worked in a facility led by a CNIO or other senior nursing informatics executive (HIMSS, 2020). Despite the increased presence of the CNIO role, our experience notes that some nurse informatics leaders exist with non-CNIO titles and many systems do not have a named *nursing informatics executive. Information from the HIMSS Workforce Survey (2020) notes that CNIOs report to a variety of other executive leaders, e.g., Chief Nurse Officers (CNOs), Chief Health Informatics Officers (CHIOs), Chief Information Officers (CIOs), etc. There is no executive-level certification exam[1] for nurse informaticists in the C-suite, and in the experience of the authors, it seems that some CNIOs serve as strategic executive partners while others live in a manager or director role that was retitled as a CNIO, without a significant shift in job duties.

---

* Attention to the certification gap was raised by Amy Rosa, DNP, RN, MSMI in a personal communication with Rebecca Freeman on March 21, 2021.

Clarity does not improve as we move out of the C-suite and into the workforce. While there *is* a certification exam for those doing the daily work of nursing informatics, there is no consistency in reporting structure or benchmarks for performance and/or value. In addition to non-standard titles and reporting structures, the HIMSS Workforce Survey (2020) underscored a variety of primary job roles for nurse informaticists in quality, implementation, development, etc. The role of a nurse informaticist can vary from an interdisciplinary team leader to a rebranded help desk staff member, possibly due to the failure to establish a national standard of work descriptions and competencies per work domain (e.g., implementation vs. development vs. quality vs. analytics, etc.) (McLane et al., 2021).

Because of the variation in titles, required educational background, job duties and reporting structures, it is often difficult to create a value proposition for a nursing informatics team. We often hear that it is difficult to quantify the value of bedside nurses with data, as well as just as difficultly explaining the work, and value of that work, in the informatics field. This seems especially true when trying to create or expand the role of nursing informatics in an organizational landscape (both operational and technical) that lags the evolution of the technological landscape itself (Ozbolt et al., 2007).

The following strategies are offered to transform this situation:

- Establish core competencies for nurse informaticists from novice to expert.
- Translate core competencies into more consistent position descriptions and career ladders opportunities.
- Create an executive informatics certification that focuses on expert-level informatics knowledge as well as executive-level leadership competencies.
- Use high-level executive competencies to more clearly define the CNIO scope and standards.
- Publish, in a central location, exemplars from large health systems where nursing informatics teams are functioning at a very high level.
- Foster informatics leaders' support of replication of best practices and successes in their own organizations.
- Establish national benchmarks to serve as measurable value and outcomes for nursing informatics.

Organizational Readiness

In many large health systems, there seems to be a lack of clarity around ownership of the health IT ecosystem. Before system-wide EHRs became widespread in hospitals and ambulatory offices, individual departments often functioned on paper or with niche applications that were largely designed and maintained by IT staff dedicated to a given area. Updates, modifications, interfaces and other strategic directions frequently were led by IT staff. As enterprise technology has come to prominence, there has been a push for operations to 'own' these systems from designating clinical champions and educators to prioritizing and designing optimization requests. In our experience, many large healthcare systems have ample opportunities to improve within this paradigm shift.

Gartner, one of the world's leading IT research and advisory companies, issued a 2018 report on successful EHR and digital care delivery programs (Gartner, 2017). Key findings support the concept of organizational readiness as a critical component of technology success:

- Success or failure of an EHR program was rarely traced to the vendor system.
- EHR and other clinical (health) IT program failures are most often traced to *inadequate organization readiness*.
- It is not unusual for CIOs and their IT organizations to focus on technology readiness when beginning an IT-related project. In doing so, it can be easy to overlook the organizational and process issues that can be *significant contributors to project failure*.
- Although clinical system implementation *should not be entirely an IT project*, CIOs are often blamed if the project experiences difficulties.

The concept of operational ownership is well-socialized with leaders in large health systems, but when asked who 'owns' any given project—the EHR, mobile technology, standalone applications—the answer often remains a member of the IT or information systems (IS) department (Jones, 2018). That reality often is reinforced by legacy frameworks of governance, where practice and technology meetings remain segregated. To move forward with a transformation of clinical (health) IT ownership, institutional leaders must urgently feel compelled to commit and implement a shared technical-operational vision of change.

There are many reasons healthcare systems *should* feel compelled to embark upon a transformation, including patient care experience and outcomes, clinician and patient engagement and satisfaction, improved margins, gains in quality, addressing workforce shortages, advancing healthcare organization partnerships, or new technology implementations. The authors have observed that smaller organizations seem to make this shift more easily. In many small institutions, one staff member may wear many hats and alignment can feel like a lighter lift. In contrast, many large health systems have complex organization charts, a significant number of staff members with matrixed reporting relationships, and a long history of institutional politics that make these paradigm shifts difficult, with few easy wins in sight.

For organizations to transform, and fully realize the role of informatics in that transformation, a health system must be ready for that transformation. Deloitte (2016) defines operational readiness as

> the structured, systematic analysis of the difference between current and future state operations, and the impact a technology implementation or optimization will have on policies, processes and roles, as well as tactics to mitigating those risks associated with adoption

and highlights that 'when effectively coordinated, operational readiness enables leaders who are best equipped to guide staff through changes, and builds capability in the organization to sustain future changes as upgrades, optimizations and new regulatory requirements are introduced' (Deloitte, 2016, p. 1). The first step toward transformation should be a strong organizational readiness assessment effort, where the facilitating team may consider the following:

- A formal organizational readiness framework.
- A compelling reason that calls for change, including a strong shared vision and credible leadership.
- Measurable process and outcome metrics that illustrate the objectives of the change.
- Engaging stakeholders across disciplines, both clinical and non-clinical. Suggested strategies to enhance organizational readiness:
  - Elevate the role of informaticists and let them lead and facilitate the redesign of frameworks for education and governance to align practice and technology.

- Empower informed ownership and organizational readiness from the executive suite to bedside staff through the role of the informaticist.
■ Readiness assessment of the organization for change and ensure an organizational readiness framework is in place; this is a separate initiative from change, technology or patient readiness.
■ *Incentivize* the operations/clinical ownership of enterprise health IT systems.
■ Begin to link the integration of technology into standard practice frameworks as part of strategic plans, variable pay/bonus structures, career advancement ladders and basic expectations to be reviewed as part of expected leadership job performance.
■ Invest in project management, ensuring that competent project managers and nurse informaticists are trained in the necessary readiness and change management frameworks, then ensure their partnership with informatics on projects, as needed.

Education

Education is one of the most difficult and multifaceted barriers to address. The historical treatment of technology as separate from practice is pervasive. Starting with the *academic setting*, nursing students must learn traditional concepts in a new way, with an understanding of technology as a core component of their practice. The AACN approved new nursing education essentials in 2021. Domain 8 provides a comprehensive starting point for informatics competencies to integrate into nursing education (AACN, 2021). However, informatics education often consists of an individual informatics class or an informatics-focused lecture series rather than being integrated into the very fabric of basic nursing education. Integration is important because nurses cannot participate in the modern practice setting at a high level if they are not prepared to utilize technology in a mature way. At the bedside, the *operational setting* also has difficulty integrating technology as a core component of nursing practice. The programs to advance nurses on the novice-to-expert continuum (Benner, 1984) often omits technology and informatics altogether. Position descriptions, clinical ladder opportunities, professional governance frameworks, nurse residency programs and other pathways to advancement in the operational domain rarely integrate informatics and technology. In terms of technology implementations and informatics, *nurse educators* and *nursing professional development specialists* often are absent partners for the informatics staff. Those roles leading the education of nursing staff should, ideally, embody the ideals of the technology/practice integration. However, the scope and standards for both positions include few references to informatics or technology. Today, there are no technology-specific competencies for the nurse educator certification and very few associated with the nursing professional development certification outline. The individuals educated and certified to assist in the academic and professional development of direct care staff have difficulty with a sense of technology ownership of systems in which they are not, themselves, proficient.

The authors have experienced a prevalent disconnect in the education area in large healthcare systems, especially as it relates to the role of the nursing informatics teams and traditional clinical educators and IT trainers. When a large healthcare system is implementing a new technology, bedside nurses should hold key roles in the evaluation, education, implementation and optimization/refinement of the technology. They should hold a role in a well-defined education framework that advances them through mature levels of technology and informatics proficiency. Superuser programs must be supported and funded with protected time for direct care staff and engage nursing operations in partnership with nursing informatics leaders who are responsible for ensuring core levels of competence in technology and analytics. Johnson (2016) emphasizes that the nursing professional development specialists of the future might be partnered with informaticists that form of partnership, making it a great first step toward engagement of the formal owners, e.g., direct care clinicians and their leaders, of any newly implemented technology.

Suggested strategies to enhance education:

■ Support key roles to operationalize the integration of technology as a core component of nursing practice by determining a path forward for:
  – *Nurse.* Informaticians must partner to support the education of faculty and, more importantly, assist faculty with the integration of technology into their existing coursework.
  – *Nurse executives.* The quality of the informatics structure for nursing staff is wholly dependent on the understanding and support of the Chief Nursing Officer (CNO). Position descriptions, clinical ladder opportunities, nurse residencies, expectations of preceptors, protected time for super users, recognition of nurse informaticists as leaders in modern-day practice start with the vision of the CNO.

– *Nurse educators and nursing professional development specialists.* There is an opportunity to update the scope and standards, and certification competencies, of both nurse educators and nursing development specialists. Leveraging the AACN Essentials (Domain 8) competencies can foster strategic alignment and ensure that position descriptions are updated.

Change Management

There are many frameworks for change management and change theory. However, in our experience, large health systems rarely identify a framework for change management and/or adhere to the basic processes when implementing health information technology. Change management is a component of organizational readiness and therefore is deserving of its own section.

In a survey of over 300 organizations, Gartner (2017) found that significant changes are the 'new normal' (Figure 8.2) for executives and staff (Gartner, 2017). Further, the impact of those changes on employee engagement is significant. For example, three planned changes negatively impact employee engagement for more than 12 months (Gartner, 2017).

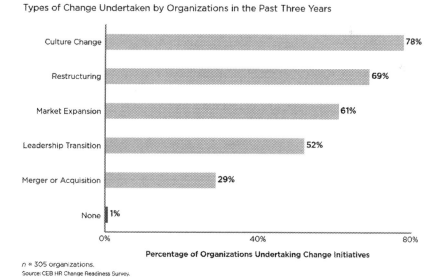

CHANGE IS THE NEW NORMAL

Types of Change Undertaken by Organizations in the Past Three Years

Culture Change — 78%
Restructuring — 69%
Market Expansion — 61%
Leadership Transition — 52%
Merger or Acquisition — 29%
None — 1%

Percentage of Organizations Undertaking Change Initiatives

n = 305 organizations.
Source: CEB HR Change Readiness Survey.

Figure 8.2   A graphical representation of the number of deaths in the Crimean War as a result of preventable infections (Nightingale F., 1858).

Optimal change management requires a dedicated, daily effort to communicate vision, maintain pressure, and engage strong sponsors/leaders. According to Meyer et al. (2018), most challenges during an implementation relate to organizational culture and suggest that efforts should be planned accordingly, preparing the clinical culture for success, and providing solutions for large-scale EHR implementation (Meyer et al., 2018). While there are expected technical challenges with change, these often are straightforward compared to the culture and change management issues. Meyer et al. (2018) recommend treating an EHR implementation as a military operation with detailed plans and timelines along with explicit roles and responsibilities.

Indeed, change management is the fulcrum for success. Prosci, Inc. (2021) describes change management as a structured process and set of tools, with a specific focus on the application of such processes where managers lead people to achieve desired outcomes amid change. These processes are within the context of both the change itself and the project management of that change (PROSCI, 2021). To the authors, there seem to be as many change management frameworks, theories and models as there are projects to which they could be applied. The selection is dependent upon organizational fit. Change initiatives fail due to many reasons, including a lack of project management framework, vision, communication, education, budget, etc. Consequently, an organization's effort to use a framework, *any framework*, is a step in the right direction. To that end, we will discuss a few key change management approaches to promote success.

Prosci® is a comprehensive, evidence-based approach to change management. The Prosci® methodology encompasses several models and includes a certification program that enables individuals in an organization to become proficient in the application of the methodology. Often considered the father of change management, Lewin (1890–1947) introduced a three-step change model (unfreeze-change-refreeze) that still accurately describes the organizational change and serves as a starting point for modern change management frameworks. Other seminal authors have written about those concepts in a more expanded way, such as Kotter, who describes an eight-stage model for understanding and managing change. Kotter (2012) refers to change management as a set of tools or structures intended to keep the change effort under control and ultimately minimize the impact on workers and avoid distractions. In their efforts to successfully implement technology, you may also see organizations referring to Rogers' 1962 diffusion of innovations theory where the term 'early adopter' originated or Norman's 1988 seven-step human–computer interaction model (Rogers, 2003 Norman, 1988). Gartner (2017) advocates for 'open source' change management where employees co-create strategy and planning and do more talking vs. 'telling' that originates above them in the leadership hierarchy (Gartner, 2017). Finally, Sittig and Singh's Socio-technical Model for Studying Health Information Technology in Complex Adaptive Healthcare Systems is a HIT-specific model of interest (Sittig & Singh, 2010). This model identifies eight unique domains that must be considered in some combination with each other when designing, implementing or evaluating a HIT initiative, including people, patients, and culture alongside the technical components of an implementation (Sittig & Singh, 2010).

While there is a need for a specific framework, it is more critical that there is a well-educated leadership team and a commitment to doing the change well. Kotter (2012) noted, 'I can't tell you how many times I've heard people use the words leadership and management synonymously and it drives me crazy' (HBR, Management is (still) Not Leadership, January 9, 2013). His sentiment was echoed by Grace Murray Hopper, one of the Navy's first female admirals, who indicated that, 'you manage things—you lead people'. We often sense this struggle within the nursing informatics community as we are frequently tasked to manage or lead *projects*, but with our expertise in technology, people and translation between the two, we should truly be driving change as leaders of practice and *people*, not just technological implementations.

Suggested strategies to address change management:

■ Adopt a formal change management approach and have change management leaders monitoring every step of the implementation.
■ Ensure the oversight of milestones and achievements of any change management framework require a dedicated effort, like project management.
■ Accept change as the new normal, shifting from the traditional top–down approach of managing change toward an open source approach involving frontline employees and consumers to co-create change strategy.
■ Ensure that nursing informatics teams have the knowledge required to lead organizations through change, to include expertise in the chosen change management framework.

A View of the Future—Our Best Nursing Informatics

In summary, the authors, with over 50 years of healthcare experience within complex healthcare organizations and large government entities. With their focus on change management and EHR implementations, the authors suggest a vision for what nursing informatics *could be*, in a large health system's drive toward organizational excellence and exemplary patient outcomes, where technology supports the best practice pathways of extraordinary care teams.

1. *The Right Team.* Are they all nurses (and if not, what do we call them)? What is their background? What is their reporting structure? How do we measure their value, and do we have national benchmarks and competencies?
2. *The Right Framework.* We live in a state of constant change—what is our roadmap for facilitating and navigating these changes, and prioritizing work, so that employees stay engaged and satisfied?
3. *Agility/Flexibility.* Everything changes—care delivery models, patient engagement tools, organizational structures, pandemics, etc. How does a nursing informatics team position itself to be highly educated, flexible, reliable, adaptable and effective?
4. *Developing Informatics Education for our Education Leaders.* Develop contemporary education offerings for both traditional faculty in academia and clinical educators in care settings, to advance their level of informatics proficiency. Engage with them in a new approach to educating nurses practicing in this modern and tech-heavy era.
5. *Advocate for more certification opportunities.* There is a need for an executive-level informatics certification—and the inclusion of informatics in other executive nursing certifications.

Nursing informatics is uniquely positioned to support an interprofessional healthcare team to facilitate healthcare transformation specifically focused on health IT systems. It is the specialty that integrates nursing science, computer science and information science to manage and communicate data, information, knowledge and wisdom into nursing practice (Saba & McCormick, 2015). In complex delivery organizations the role of the nurse informatics executive is expanding. The executive nurse informaticist combines knowledge of evidence-based practice, change management, leadership, nursing care and technology expertise. This unique set of skills is imperative to the success of organizations seeking to find value in new health IT delivery systems. Consequently, healthcare organizations developing interdisciplinary teams must include nurse informatics as a key member to maximize value and help the organization solve system-level problems.

Further, a CNIO as part of the executive team is essential in assuring quality. As Deming (2014) reminds us:

> Hard work will not ensure quality. Best efforts will not ensure quality, and will neither gadgets, computers nor investment in machinery. A necessary ingredient for improvement of quality is the application of profound knowledge. There is no substitute for knowledge. Knowledge we have in abundance. We must learn to use it.

(Edwards Deming, 2014, p. 38)

Research has reported work environments of nurses are characterized by a high workload, time pressures, lack of leadership support, inadequate organization governance and increasing burden of EHRs, which leads to turnover, job dissatisfaction and burnout (Boyle et al., 2019). The coronavirus pandemic and mobilization of healthcare forces have pushed the optimization of EHRs and other health technologies; these efforts uncovered efficiency opportunities and highlighted CNIOs and nurse informaticists as essential team leaders and operational partners. As Boyle (date) asserts by implementing true interprofessional teams, joy in work will be restored by fostering a connectedness and true interprofessional collaborative practice. Furthermore, leveraging the roles of all team members increases respect and partnerships. An interprofessional team that includes informatics nursing leadership helps to inform the design of health IT and EHRs. We believe that usability issues are well-documented issues, and given EHRs were not designed with nursing documentation as a priority, it is understandable that nurses are frustrated addressing EHR issues.

Finally, the implementation of a health IT solution is not a one-time change transformation effort. Advancing health IT implementation, adoption and usability through blended teams is foundational to all healthcare transformation efforts. More than a decade ago, the goals set forth by the U.S. Department of Health and Human Services established financial incentives for the adoption of EHRs. The expectation of health IT implementation and adoption was to solve healthcare deficiencies and provide tools for clinicians with the goal of interoperability and improved outcomes. Today, leaders are struggling with the challenges of health IT usability and clinician burnout. In fact, for many, the EHR is seen as an obstacle instead of an asset (Gettinger & Zayas-Cabán, 2021). The key to improvements in safety, effectiveness, and efficiency of EHRs, and ultimately patient care is to focus on the daily work of direct care clinicians supported by leadership (IHI, 2016). Leadership commitment at the most senior level is necessary to cultivate and lead clinical and technical improvements throughout the healthcare system. Excellent health delivery demands health IT capability to support clinical skills and continuously improve the systems. Deming (2014) described a 'system' as a set of interdependent structures, people and processes working together, harnessing the power of genuine collaboration is essential for high performing systems, Deming's overriding message: quality and operations are all about the system, not individual performance. The system has to be designed so the worker can perform well (Orsini, 2013). Nursing informaticists and CNIOs are key team members prepared to lead these transformations.

References

AACN. (2021). *The New 1. AACN essentials*. Available at: https://www.aacnnursing.org/AACN-Essentials (Accessed: 26 December 2021).

American Nurses Association, ed. (2014). *Nursing informatics: Scope and standards of practice*. 2nd ed. Silver Spring, MD: American Nurses Association.

Benner, P. (1984). *From novice to expert, excellence, and power in clinical nursing practice*. Menlo Park, CA: Addison-Wesley Publishing Company, p.307.

Boyle, D. K., Baernholdt, M., Adams, J. M., McBride, S., Harper, E., Poghosyan, L., & Manges, K. (2019). Improve nurses' well-being and joy in work: Implement true interprofessional teams and address electronic health record usability issues. *Nursing Outlook*, 67(6), pp.791–797.

Brown, S. H. et al. (2003). VistA - U.S. Department of Veterans Affairs national-scale HIS. *International Journal of Medical Informatics*, pp.135–156. https://doi.org/10.1016/S1386-5056(02)00131-4

Cummins, M., Gundlapalli, A., Murray, P., Park, H.-A. & Lehmann, C. (2016). Nursing informatics certification worldwide: History, pathway, roles and motivation. *Yearbook of Medical Informatics*, 2016(1), pp.264–271. Available at: https://www.ncbi.nlm.nih.gov/pmc/articles/PMC5171559/ (Accessed: 3 July 2021).

Deckro, J., Phillips, T., Davis, A., Hehr, A. T. & Ochylski, S. (2021). Big data in the veterans health administration: A nursing informatics perspective. *Journal of Nursing Scholarship*, 53(3), pp.288–295.

Deming, W. E. (2014). *Understanding profound knowledge* [online]. Available at: https://deming.org/too-many-people-putting-forth-their-best-efforts/ (Accessed 13 September 2021).

Gartner, Inc. (2017). Available at: https://www.gartner.com/en/documents/3825770/open-source-change-making-change-management-work (Accessed 11 August 2021).

Gettinger, A. & Zayas-Cabán, T. (2021). HITECH to 21st century cures: Clinician burden and evolving health IT policy. *Journal of the American Medical Informatics Association*, 28(5), pp.1022–1025.

Health Information Management and Systems Society. (2020). *2020 Nursing informatics workforce survey*. Available at: https://www.himss.org/sites/hde/files/media/file/2020/05/15/himss_nursinginformaticssurvey2020_v4.pdf (Accessed 29 July 2021).

Health Information Management and Systems Society. (2021). *Job mine: Informaticist*. Available at: https://jobmine.himss.org/jobs/?keywords=informaticist&pos_flt=0&location=&location_completion=&location_type=&location_text=&location_autocomplete=true (Accessed 11 July 2021).

Jackson, T. & Ross, H. (2019). *From tactician to strategist: The evolving role of the CNIO | healthsystemcio.com* (no date). Available at: https://healthsystemcio.com/2019/05/13/from-tactician-to-strategist-the-evolving-role-of-the-cnio/ (Accessed: 26 December 2021).

Johnson, J. A. (2016). Nursing professional development specialists of the future. *Journal for Nurses in Professional Development*, 32(3), pp.158–160. https://doi.org/10.1097/NND.0000000000000251

Jones, M. (2018). *Organizational readiness is key to successful EHR and digital care delivery programs*. Stamford, CT: Gartner, Inc. 25 Jan 2018, ID G00349780.

Kotter, J. P. (2012). *Leading change*. Boston, MA: Harvard Business Press, p.194.

Lewin, K. (1947). Frontiers in group dynamics: Concept, method and reality in social science; equilibrium and social change. *Human Relations*, 1(1), pp.5–41.

McLane, T. M., Hoyt, R., Hodge, C., Weinfurter, E., Reardon, E. E. & Monsen, K. A. (2021). What industry wants: an empirical analysis of health informatics job postings. *Applied Clinical Informatics*, 12(2), pp.285–292.

Meyer, G. S., O'Neil, B., & Gross, D. (2018). Seven challenges and seven solutions for large-scale EHR Implementations. *NEJM Catalyst*, 4(5). Available at: https://catalyst.nejm.org/doi/full/10.1056/CAT.18.0073

Murphy, J. (2011). The nursing informatics workforce: who are they and what do they do? *Nursing Economics*, 29(3), pp.150–154.

Nightingale, F. (1858). Figure 8.1: Diagram of the causes of mortality in the army in the east. *From notes on matters affecting the health, efficiency, and hospital administration of the british army*. https://www.florence-nightingale.co.uk/wp-content/uploads/t5.jpg

Norman, D. (1988). *The psychology of everyday things*. New York: Basic Books, p.257.

Office of the National Coordinator for Health IT. (2017). Percent of hospitals, by type, that possess certified health IT. Available at: https://dashboard.heal thit.gov/quickstats/pages/certified-electronic-health-record-technology-in-hospi-tals.php (Accessed 3 July 2021).

Orsini, J. N. (2013). *Essential deming: Leadership principles from the father of qual-ity*. London: McGraw-Hill Education, p.336.

Ozbolt, J., Faimbe, E. S. N., Roberts, D. & Wilson, M. (2007). How about a career in nursing informatics?. *American Nurse*. Available at: https://www.myamerican-nurse.com/how-about-a-career-in-nursing-informatics/ (Accessed 30 August 2021).

Ozbolt, J. G. & Saba, V. K. (2008). A brief history of nursing informatics in the United States of America. *Nursing Outlook*, 56(5), pp.199–205.

Prosci, Inc. (2021). What is change management? Retrieved July 17, 2021 from https://www.prosci.com/resources/articles/what-is-change-management

Rogers, E. M. (2003). *Diffusion of innovations*. 5th ed. Free Press, p.512.

Saba, V. K., & McCormick, K. A. (2015). *Essentials of nursing informatics*. 6th ed. London: McGraw-Hill Education, p.886.

Scoville, R., Little, K., Rakover, J., Luther, K. & Mate, K. (2016). *Sustaining improve-ment*. IHI White Paper. Cambridge, MA: Institute for Healthcare Improvement. Available at: ihi.org (Accessed 30 August 2021).

Sittig, D. F., & Singh, H. (2010). A new sociotechnical model for studying health information technology in complex adaptive healthcare systems. *Quality & Safety in Health Care. NIH Public Access*, 19 Suppl 3(Suppl 3), p.i68. https://doi.org/10.1136/qshc.2010.042085

Szpaichler, S., Drake, N. & Reichbach, C. (2016). Driving impact through opera-tional readiness: Operational preparation for enabling technology transforma-tion in health care. Deloitte Development, LLC. Available at: https://www2.deloitte.com/content/dam/Deloitte/us/Documents/life-sciences-health-care/us-lshc-operational-readiness.pdf (Accessed 9 August 2021).

Chapter 9

Nursing Informatics within Health Systems: Global Comparison

Fabio D'Agostino, Miriam de Abreu Almeida,
Aline Tsuma Gaedke Nomura and Jude L. Tayaben

Contents

DOI: 10.4324/9781003054849-9

Using Clinical Nursing Information Systems to Predict Healthcare Outcomes: An Italian Experience

A clinical nursing information system (CNIS) is an integrated, computer-assisted system designed to store, manipulate and retrieve information concerned with the clinical aspects of providing nursing care within different healthcare settings (Liaskos & Mantas, 2002). Within electronic health records (EHRs), CNISs can be implemented since EHRs should contain information about care encounters between healthcare providers (e.g., physicians, nurses) and patients (Ambinder, 2005). However, EHRs often do not allow or support the ability to store, manipulate or retrieve information about nursing care due to a poor design and a lack of a set of minimum nursing care elements such as the Nursing Minimum Data Set (Lytle et al., 2021; Werley et al., 1991). In order to address this issue, a research project was started in Italy in 2010 with the aim of developing and implementing a CNIS and, later, evaluating its impact by using nursing-generated data (D'Agostino et al., 2013). This project was developed by the doctoral program in Nursing Science at the Department of Biomedicine at Tor Vergata University and funded by the Italian Center of Excellence for Nursing Scholarship, Rome, Italy (D'Agostino, 2014).

The PAI System

The CNIS, called Professional Assessment Instrument (PAI) system, was developed in two years (D'Agostino et al., 2012). The PAI system originates from a similar but different system (the PAI-UDI) that was already in place in another healthcare setting (i.e., a community nursing-led unit) (Zega et al., 2010). The PAI system allows the collection of nursing care data according to the nursing process. Structured and standard data, such as nursing assessment data, nursing diagnoses, nursing interventions and outcomes and unstructured data, such as nursing notes, are recorded by nurses through the PAI system (D'Agostino et al., 2019b). A PAI built-in clinical decision support system supports nurses in their choice of nursing diagnoses and interventions. The clinical decision support system was validated by a team of experts (Zega et al., 2014).

Before its implementation, the PAI system was pilot tested for three months in a hospital. Subsequently, the PAI was registered with the Italian Society of Authors and Publishers as a computer program. It is owned by the Nursing Board of Rome, Italy and is a royalty-free software (D'Agostino, 2014).

The PAI system has been implemented at the A. Gemelli hospital in Rome, Italy (1,500 beds) since 2013 as an integral part of the EHR of the hospital and is used by nurses to record their care (D'Agostino et al., 2017).

Care data collected daily by nurses using the PAI system can also be used for secondary purposes such as research. A literature review highlighted that standard nursing data such as nursing diagnoses can predict different patient and organizational outcomes such as length of stay, costs, mortality, quality of life, amount of nursing care, discharge dispositions, sleep quality, glycemic control in different healthcare settings (Sanson et al., 2017).

Descriptive Studies Using Nursing-generated Data Collected by the PAI System

An early study conducted with data collected by the PAI system showed that standard nursing data, such as nursing diagnoses, were able to describe patients with different care complexities among several different medical conditions. This complexity was associated with hospital length of stay and mortality (D'Agostino et al., 2017). Another study provided a description of nursing care delivered in an oncology department. Through the use of a nursing minimum data set generated by the PAI system, findings show that most nursing interventions were delivered based on a nursing prescription and not on a medical order (Sanson et al., 2019a). In another study, data generated by the PAI-UDI (e.g., nursing diagnoses and interventions) was used to describe the care delivered by nurses in a community nursing-led unit. Results highlighted different medical and nursing needs of this population compared to hospitalized acute patients (Zeffiro et al., 2018).

Predictive Models Using Nursing-generated Data Collected by the PAI System

Two retrospective studies were conducted to predict hospital length of stay and mortality, respectively, using data collected by the PAI system and the hospital discharge register over a period of six months (D'Agostino et al., 2019a; Sanson et al., 2019b). The aim was to predict the length of stay and length of stay deviation (i.e., the difference between the actual length of stay and the DRG-specific national expected hospital length of stay) (D'Agostino et al., 2019a). Nursing diagnoses collected on admission, patients' sociodemographic data (age, gender), clinical conditions (i.e., the All Patient Refined-Diagnosis Related Group (APR-DRG) weight, the Charlson comorbidity index), and organizational data (admitting inpatient unit, modality of admission) were used as predictors. A sample of 2,190 consecutively admitted patients in four inpatient units (two medical and two surgical) of the study hospital were included. Two least-squares multiple linear regression models were performed to test the association between nursing diagnoses and length of stay and length of stay deviation after controlling for the above-mentioned predictors. In both models, nursing diagnoses were an independent predictor of length of stay and length of stay deviation. Moreover, nursing diagnoses were one of the few independent predictors of the length of stay deviation jointly with gender and modality of admission the only variable related to patient conditions, which could be described from a medical (e.g., medical diagnosis) as well as nursing (e.g., nursing diagnosis) perspective.

The second study aimed to predict hospital mortality in a sample of 2,301 medical and surgical patients using the following variables: the nursing dependency index (NDI) as expressed by the number of nursing diagnoses on admission, gender, age, the APR-DRG weight, the Charlson comorbidity index and the modality of admission (Sanson et al., 2019b). Eight logistic regression models were used starting from a basic model (Model 1) with age, gender and modality of admission as predictors. Then seven models were tested, adding to the first model the following variables: the NDI (Model 2), the Charlson comorbidity index (Model 3), the APR-DRG weight (Model 4), the Charlson comorbidity index and the NDI (Model 5), the NDI and the APR-DRG weight (Model 6), the Charlson comorbidity index and the APR-DRG weight (Model 7), and the Charlson comorbidity index, the NDI and the APR-DRG weight (Model 8).

The number of nursing diagnoses on admission was an independent predictor of hospital mortality. Moreover, when nursing diagnoses were added to the model the variance increased by 20%. Model 8. The addition of nursing diagnoses was highly accurate (with a c statistic = 0.89, 95% confidence interval: 0.87–0.92); the bootstrapping method also showed the internal validity of the model.

Predictive Model Using Nursing-generated Data Collected by the PAI-UDI

A retrospective study was conducted to identify the predictors of a longer length of stay in a community nursing-led unit (Zeffiro et al., 2020). A sample of 904 patients consecutively admitted in a community nursing-led unit

(15 beds) over a period of seven years was enrolled. Nursing diagnoses on admission (total number and specific diagnoses), nursing interventions, the Barthel index; sociodemographic (gender, age and marital status), organizational (modality of admission and of discharge) variables and clinical conditions (the APR-DRG weight, the Charlson comorbidity index) were used as predictors. A backward stepwise logistic regression was performed to estimate the association between the above predictors and a prolonged length of stay. The number of nursing diagnoses, specific nursing diagnoses and nursing interventions were found to be independent predictors of a prolonged length of stay. Conversely, other nursing interventions were shown to be independent predictors of a lower length of stay.

Italian Perspective Conclusion

CNISs are essential to describe the nursing care delivered, patients' conditions and outcomes, costs incurred and for management, organizational and research purposes. The results of these studies have shown that nursing-generated data are useful predictors for healthcare outcomes in different healthcare settings in addition to commonly used variables (e.g., coded medical diagnoses and interventions, sociodemographic data).

To our knowledge, in Italy, the use of systems like the PAI and PAI-UDI is unique, even though the use of standard nursing terminologies (one of the prerequisites of a CNIS) is increasing (Mazzoleni et al., 2018). It is reasonable to expect implementations of new systems to occur in shorter periods. Interestingly, the Nursing Informatics Italian Group (NIIG) has been constituted in 2021within the Italian Nurses Association called CNAI (National Association of Nurses Associations) (CNAI-HIMSS Gruppo Italiano Nursing Informatics, 2021). The aim of the NIIG is to improve the role of nurse informaticians recognizing it as a specialty in Italy and providing expertise in this field through research, educational, networking and partnership activities. The NIIG is linked with the Italian International Classification for Nursing Practice (ICNP) Research & Development Centre, which has an official partnership with the Healthcare Information and Management Systems Society (HIMSS) (Italian ICNP Research & Development Centre, 2021).

Moreover, since the PAI system is a royalty-free software package, the agreement with other healthcare institutions can easily be achieved to promote the use of a CNIS in EHRs. Notably, a modified version of the PAI system will be implemented in the context of the family and community nurse program in the Lazio Region (Savini et al., 2021).

The spread of systems like the PAI, which also enables easy retrieval and analyses of data, can promote the continuity of care that is supported by a consistent flow of minimum information about the patients' healthcare status within different healthcare settings. Indeed, health policy choices should be guided by comprehensive information about the care provided (e.g., medical and nursing care) and population health needs (D'Agostino et al., 2012).

A Brazilian Nursing Information System Perspective

Brazil has about 212 million inhabitants, comprising 5,570 municipalities distributed in 26 states (IBGE, 2021). With the sixth largest population and occupying the fifth position in territorial extension in the world (IBGE, 2021), Brazil has demonstrated its initiative in promoting national and international big data policies (Mahrenbach et al., 2018). Among the Brazilian initiatives in data science, the Brazilian support networks GO FAIR Brasil and the Brazilian Open Data Portal stand out (Brasil, 2018a, 2021). The FAIR principles, an acronym for Findable, Accessible, Interoperable and Reusable, are recognized worldwide as key elements for good practice in all data management processes. The objective of both is to make all types of data, which are fragmented and disconnected, more easily located, accessible, interoperable and reusable, seeking the development of a shared global environment focused on data-based research and innovation in health. Today, GO FAIR Brasil-Saúde is the first active implementation network in operation, serving as a model for other areas, such as agriculture, nuclear and digital humanities, which are in the process of negotiating access (Brasil, 2021).

Considering the strengths and weaknesses of Brazil in terms of the digital age, seven digital health strategies were planned to be established and developed between 2019 and 2023. The first strategy ensures the Ministry of Health governance leadership can rely on the active collaboration of external actors; the second targets implementing and expanding health informatics at all levels of care; the third offers support to care delivery with the integration of telehealth and digital services into the assistance workflow; the fourth develops actions for greater involvement of users and health professionals; the fifth proposes to promote managers and health professionals training, as well as for information technology professionals; the sixth seeks to promote interoperability between health services; while the seventh strategy aims to expand the services of the national health data network, including the implementation of electronic prescription and development of health surveillance initiatives. In addition, emphasis is placed on developing initiatives in the Internet of Things, with remote monitoring and diagnostics, use of mobile terminals with access to medical databases and enabling electronic medical records and big data and secondary use of data (Brasil, 2021; Brazil, 2018a).

Like other developing countries, public health has always been a challenge in Brazil. In order to promote health in a universal, egalitarian and participatory way, the Unified Health System (SUS) was instituted in 1988 under the Brazilian Constitution. Two years later, the construction of the National Health Information System (SNIS) aimed to establish a fully integrated health system in the country. Since then, several investments have been made in this direction, but none has been effectively implemented throughout the nation (Brasil, 2016).

However, in 2013 the Brazilian Government started the implementation of e-SUS APS (computerization of Primary Care Strategy), a qualified computerization process in search for an electronic SUS. This system has two software components: System with Simplified Data Collection (CDS) and the Citizen Electronic Health Record System (PEC) (Brasil, 2020). The PEC allows the construction of a database with all the patient's personal and clinical information, stored during the encounter in order to computerize the flow of the citizen in the healthcare system (Brasil, 2020). This tool is an instrument that is used daily by health professionals, including nurses (Gomes et al., 2019).

Nurses play an important role in the Brazilian management of public health services (Clara et al., 2020). The nurse, as the care manager, is one of the main professionals responsible for the consolidation of the data. The care provided to people, families and the community, as well as the care documentation in the health record, is regulated by the Federal Council of Nursing. The Federal Council of Nursing established the use of the nursing process (NP) as a method to systematize nursing care in Brazil (Hermida, 2010). The NP, in its five stages, must be carried out deliberately and systematically in all public or private environments where there is professional nursing care (Conselho Federal de Enfermagem, 2009). The computerization of this process is pointed out as a solution, as it proposes to qualify the formulation and execution of the nursing process; thus, effectively consolidating the surveillance to improve the quality of health processes (Clara et al., 2020). With the automation and qualification of information management systems, the work process and care practices are consequently strengthened.

Health information supports the decision-making of professionals and managers for the actions of care, control and social participation in Brazil

(Meirelles & Cunha, 2020). The SUS Computer Department (DATASUS) was created with the objective of computerizing SUS activities, including electronic health records. Its mission is to provide information systems and computer support (Meirelles & Cunha, 2020). DATASUS is responsible for managing the Health Information Systems (SIS), which allow the collection, processing, analysis and dissemination of information (Grasiely et al., 2020), and the internal management systems of the Ministry of Health (Meirelles & Cunha, 2020). DATASUS is the classic example of big data (Stelmach & Cruz, 2017), and although research is being developed from this perspective, it is seldom explored by researchers (Costi et al., 2017; Stelmach & Cruz, 2017).

Regarding authenticity and digital preservation of electronic records in health, the Personal Data Protection law is the first Brazilian policy to establish specific rules for the treatment of personal information for research in order to maintain the privacy and confidentiality of personal data, including considering the anonymization of such data (Brasil, 2018b).

From a hospital perspective, the sharing and reuse of information between electronic health systems is a major challenge, given the non-existence of a standard language capable of covering all available health domains in electronic health records (Park et al., 2011). As hospital clinical data in Brazil is not organized in a single repository, it is difficult for researchers to find common terms of interest. These characteristics have a substantial impact on pre-processing requirements, quality of linked data and internal validity of the search results from the data (Kharrat et al., 2020; Lacerda et al., 2020; Sanni Ali et al., 2019).

Information technology combined with the Computerized Nursing Process has been considered an efficient strategy for improvements in nursing care. This approach optimizes accurate and complete information for the care unit, providing fast information contained in the medical record for the multidisciplinary team, in addition to systematizing the work and promoting patient safety (Paese et al., 2018).

The Standardized Language Systems (SLP) used in the diagnosis, interventions and nursing outcomes stages offer a conceptual framework that facilitates the documentation of the NP and aids in clinical reasoning and decision-making about patient care. SLPs are considered a prerequisite for the construction of EHR, enabling the retrieval of information for research, statistical analysis, big data, among others. The SLP most used by Brazilian nurses are NANDA International (NANDA-I) for the nursing diagnoses, Nursing Outcomes Classification (NOC), Nursing Interventions Classification (NIC) and ICNP (De Oliveira & Peres, 2021; Rabelo-Silva et al., 2017).

A successful example in a hospital management system, Management Application for University Hospitals (AGHU), with a focus on the patient, was adopted as a standard for all federal university hospitals affiliated to the Brazilian Company of Hospital Services (Ebserh), a state company linked to the Ministry of Education (MEC). The application aims to support the standardization of care and administrative practices in hospitals and to allow the creation of national indicators in order to facilitate the creation of common improvement programs for all these units (Ministério da Educação, 2020).

To develop AGHU, Ebserh used as a foundation the Hospital Management Application (AGH), a system developed in a university hospital in the south of the country, taking into account the success of its management model (Ministério da Educação, 2020). This project enabled the hospital to migrate and update the old AGH to the current AGHUse system, transforming an internal solution into a comprehensive, modern and registered platform with a general public license. Thus, AGHUse became a free software, generating results that move toward transforming the reality of healthcare management in the country, disseminated to six important hospital companies, including the Air Force and the Brazilian Army (HCPA, 2020; Ministério da Educação, 2020). Thus, the use of the same electronic system, with similar evolution in these scenarios, allows the creation of a single repository that includes clinical, administrative and demographic information for the country.

Although this is not a reality for the entire national territory, the AGHUse offers many research possibilities due to its immense database. The electronic patient record is one of its modules; it contains documentation from health professionals, including the nursing process performed for all hospitalized patients, as well as the outpatient nursing consultation. Recent and innovative research in the nursing field was the development of an information model (IM) on pain management, based on Hospital de Clínicas de Porto Alegre (HCPA) big data, an institution accredited by the Joint Commission International (JCI) (Nomura et al., 2018, 2021). The data science methodology used allowed management of all data extracted from EHRs of patients admitted to clinical and surgical units for five years. Based on this IM, it is possible to optimize the electronic health system, improve qualifying of the patient care delivery in pain management, in addition to presenting potential for its use in predictive modeling (Nomura et al., 2021, 2021). In the HCPA, nurses document patient care in the electronic health record using the NANDA-I and NIC classifications. In addition, research on the clinical applicability of the NOC has been developed based on data collected on this computerized platform (Nabinger et al., 2020; Pires et al., 2020). This research strengthens the effectiveness of the care provided by nurses.

Considering the context of digital health, telemedicine is extremely relevant in Brazil due to the large territory containing rural areas and remote territories with scarce health resources and gaps in healthcare. This technology has expanded to progressively assist in health, research and education. Telemedicine entered the country in 1990 in a fragmented way, and after 2011 public administrative initiatives started the process of integrating this sector along with SUS. In 2018 it was named digital health. However, the Brazilian telemedicine policy is still in the process of development (Silva et al., 2020).

Telehealth received important support with the advent of COVID-19. Among the digital strategies used to improve these public health strategies in this context, telehealth generated a great deal of movement in Brazil (Caetano et al., 2020). This technology provided capabilities for remote screening, care and treatment, aid in monitoring, surveillance, detection and prevention of healthcare indirectly related to COVID-19, strengthening the unique and universal health system in Brazil (Caetano et al., 2020).

Thus, digital health is changing the way nurses deliver patient care. The processes by which nurses make clinical decisions, communicate with patients and their families, and implement clinical interventions are and will continue to be modified. However, to qualify for nursing work through digital health, it is necessary for nurses to develop specific skills in the digital area (Barbosa et al., 2021). In Brazil, there are few leaders and educators with skills in nursing digital health (Barbosa, 2017). Among the critical areas of education in the country, nursing informatics stands out. Although the importance of this competence is broad and involves the effective management of information collected from the patient to assist in decision-making, incorporation of this discipline is rare in Brazilian curricula. Thus, it is necessary to expand skills via training in undergraduate and graduate nursing courses, continuing education programs and professional education initiatives. Furthermore, the opportunity to develop these skills can extend beyond formal academia and connect with ongoing professional development international networks and programs (Barbosa, 2017).

Brazilian Perspective Conclusion

Although the challenges are many, health technologies in Brazil will benefit from such institutional and technological advances in data processing and analysis to produce evidence on the cost, effectiveness and safety of health technologies, as well as their impact on social, economic and health policies. In this context, it is relevant that Brazilian nurses take decision-making positions at different levels of healthcare. They must be prepared for these positions with adequate knowledge based on scientific evidence.

The Philippine Perspectives: Overview of eHealth in the Philippines

Three decades ago eHealth started to progress in the Philippines. In 1998, the National Telehealth Center was born at the University of the Philippines Manila. The center is the leading research unit inside the University of the Philippines responsible for developing cost-effective tools and innovations in the realm of information and communications technology (ICT) for improving healthcare. One year later, a study group was called for the development of Standards for Health Information, aiming to determine standards for health information in the country.

In early 2000, eHealth was then recognized for its relevance as a support system for the improvement of health ICT infrastructure towards better health outcomes. The Department of Health (DOH) published the National Objectives for Health, 2005–2010 and 2011–2016, prioritized the use of ICT in various reform areas, critical health programs and specific areas in health administration. In 2014, the Philippines eHealth Strategic Framework and Plan (PeHSFP) was released and describes how the eHealth vision will be achieved to guide national coordination and collaboration, and sets clear direction and guidance to the ongoing and future eHealth activities in the country. The major sections of the framework were eHealth in the context of the Philippines, strategic framework, action plan, and monitoring and evaluation (Department of Health & Department of Science and Technology (DOST), 2014).

The DOH defined eHealth as a tool concerned with improving the flow of information, through electronic means, to support and facilitate the delivery of quality and responsive health services, and better management of health systems and service delivery networks. It is envisioned that,

> By 2020, eHealth will enable widespread access to healthcare services, health information, and securely share and exchange client's information in support to a safer, quality healthcare, more equitable

and responsive health system for all the Filipino people by transforming the way information is used to plan, manage, deliver and monitor health services.

(DOH & DOST, 2014)

Though challenging to achieve this vision, the Department of Health released relevant circulars and guidelines up to the present. Such guidelines gave directions as to how eHealth would be managed and implemented to address informatics and health inequities in the country.

Several innovations were developed by the leading higher education institutions, supported by the DOH, and also by non-government organizations to address community and clinical issues using digital health facilities and applications. Notable projects include the Community Health Information Tracking System (CHITS), RxBox, e-HATID and Wireless for Health platform, to name a few. In 2005, the University of the Philippines Manila started to offer the Master of Science in Health Informatics (MSHI). It is the only informatics program offered in the country. Accordingly, students enrolled are expected to implement the principles and concepts of health information system development within an existing environment relevant to their practice. To expand its network, the Philippines is an active member of the Asian eHealth Informatics Network (AeHIN) that was launched to strengthen digital health initiatives in South and Southeast Asian countries. This network is composed of a pool of health and IT professionals committed to promote better use of ICTs to achieve better health (AeHIN, 2011).

With the transformation of eHealth infrastructure led by the DOH and other institutions, we now see the developments of relevant innovations and improved medical and health practice as we experience these both in the community and hospitals across the country. Indeed, the eHealth system in the Philippines is progressing dramatically, now that different professionals such as nurses, midwives and other higher education institutions are actively engaged in ensuring informatics is used in various settings, such as teaching to the academia and improvement of practice in the community, and the importance of digital health toward achieving better health outcomes as a whole.

History of Nursing Informatics in the Philippines

Sumabat (2010) mentioned that nursing informatics started when the Philippine Nurses Association (PNA), the accredited national nurses' organization in the Philippines, participated in the development of Standards for Health Information in the Philippines (SHIP) in 1999. Later in 2010, the Philippine Nursing Informatics Association (PNIA) was formed, and in 2012, the Informatics Nurses Society of the Philippines (INurseSP) as the sub-specialty organization of PNA for nursing informatics and accredited by the Professional Regulation Commission. INurseSP is the official Philippine representative to the International Medical Informatics Association- Nursing Informatics Special Interest Group (INurseSP, 2017). Despite two Associations in nursing informatics, the nurses' role and functions are not clear yet. However, we noticed active participation of nurses in some eHealth initiatives in the country, including Telehealth in nursing. According to Bernal et al. (2008), with Telehealth, as an alternative medium to address healthcare needs in geographically isolated areas through the use of information and communication technology, nurses provide care for patients or populations through electronic communication media and act as triage nurses who advise and consult with patients and clients. The National Telehealth Center in Manila is ensuring that telehealth nurses are attending training and seminars, and they are in vanguard to promote telehealth nursing in the Philippines as one of the latest specializations in nursing. In 2009, nursing informatics started to be offered as one additional course in the Bachelor of Science in Nursing in lieu of the Basics in Computer, now offered in senior high school.

Use of Information Technology in Clinical and Community Practice

Notable clinical and community-based innovations already implemented in the country are Community Health Information Tracking System (CHITS), RxBOX, eHealth Tablet for Informed Decision Making of LGUs (eHATID), and Wireless Access for Health (WAH). According to the National Institute of Health, CHITS is the first electronic medical record (EMR) system for government-based health facilities certified by the Philippine Health Insurance and widely used at the Regional Health Unit (RHU) level. This has reduced patients' waiting time and improved monitoring of patient care through efficient data encoding and records retrieval. The Philippine Council of Health Research and Development is proud that this technology aims to contribute to the effective and efficient delivery of health services through appropriate information and communication strategy. It can aid in health decision-making at the local level through patient's records searching requiring only a few seconds upon admission, and laboratory requests, results and reports can be generated automatically.

The RxBox is a multi-component program (biomedical device, electronic medical record system and telemedicine training) designed to provide better access to life-saving healthcare services in isolated and disadvantaged communities nationwide. It is an ICT innovation designed to support the Department of Health's call for *Kalusugan Pangkalahatan* or Universal Health Care.

The eHATID is one of the eHealth and Community Empowerment through Science and Technology (CEST) projects of the Philippine Council for Health Research and Development (PCHRD) of the Department of Science and Technology (DOST) with Ateneo De Manila University. Accordingly, the subsystems of this are (1) EMR for efficient patient data management; (2) eHATID LGU Dashboard for real-time visualization of local patients for decision-making of the LGU; and (3) Mayor-Doctor Communication as a channel for decision-making and sharing of health-related information.

The WAH is an open-source health management information system (HMIS) software developed specifically for local governments and community health facilities. It is validated by PhilHealth, endorsed by the Department of Health, and adheres to the Health and Primary Care Provider Network requirements of the Universal Health Care law. The products of WAH are anchored on the needs of clinics, hospitals, patients and even the COVID-19 risk assessment, monitoring and management system, and these are being availed by the municipal and community-based clinics and hospitals in the country.

Nursing Informatics in Education

NI started in the nursing education in the Philippines when the Commission on Higher Education Memorandum Order (CMO) 14, series of 2009 included informatics as one course in the Bachelor of Science in Nursing curriculum. The course deals with the use of information technology systems and data standards based on nursing informatics principles/theories. It further guides the utilization of clinical information systems in the management and decision-making of patient care.

The World Health Organization (WHO, 2010) argued that the capabilities of Filipino nurses are most affected by the nursing education delivered in more than 450 nursing programs to over 500,000 students nationwide. The Commission on Higher Education (CHED) has recognized the need for nursing schools to increase the overall quality of nursing graduates, and to that end is encouraging and tracking the increased use of informatics in nursing programs. The wider use of informatics in nursing curricula is seen as essential to improving the quality of the nursing education that schools are delivering (WHO, 2010). With this call, nursing schools started to procure e-learning facilities as additional learning and teaching modality with the use of videos and demonstration models. Another support for e-Learning is high simulation models used in the skills laboratory and virtual hospital. Schools have also started to explore online open access books and journals, and others.

Recent CMO 15, series of 2017 of the Bachelor of Science in Nursing strengthened the NI course, and the Living in the IT Era included an elective course (CMO, 2017). The course deals with concepts, principles, theories and techniques on NI in clinical practice, education and research. The learners are expected to use the informatics system to support healthcare delivery. Thus, the related learning experiences or skills demonstrations require students to at least develop competencies to website development, use of statistics and qualitative data analysis applications, advanced Microsoft use in infographics development, and creation of mobile applications applicable for community-based health programs. To increase the capacity of nursing instructors, the Association of Deans of the Philippine Colleges of Nursing (ADPCN) through Philippine Nursing Education Academy (PNEA) spearheaded training and workshops in teaching NI. Last year, they published online the compilation of best practices on Related Learning Experience (RLE) alternative learning. We have experienced how we could maximize informatics use in nursing education, practice and research, especially this time of the pandemic.

Nursing Informatics in Research

Recent developments in nursing research are quite limited. For more than ten years of NI in the curriculum, the Philippines doesn't have any notable research activities and outputs related to digital health and nursing. However, collaborative studies have been conducted with the International Medical Informatics Association-Nursing Informatics group. However, interesting NI topics that need investigation are the following: relevant NI agenda, AI in nursing and impact of remote learning, flexible learning and simulation in nursing education, using and development of research methods, among others. The undergraduate research course should expand in NI studies using appropriate NI methods, theories and frameworks. Related theories and emerging frameworks widely used in the Philippine nursing and health informatics studies are the Technological Competency as Caring in Nursing (Locsin & Purnell, 2015); Unified Theory of Acceptance and Use of Technology (Venkatesh et al., 2003); Davis Technology Acceptance Model; and e-Learning self-efficacy. The research introduced as a method has moved to venture development of mobile applications, online e-learning materials and other related online facilities. Using models, frameworks and research guided Filipino nursing students to develop self-monitoring mobile applications that can be used by patients with diabetes mellitus, one assessment app to be used by healthcare providers for older persons in the community, and another one to profile the mood status of students.

Challenges and Future Directions of NI in the Philippines

Though nursing informatics is widely recognized as a course and integrated into the BSN curriculum and active participation of nurses in eHealth, and relevant studies have been conducted, several key challenges have been identified. Using these challenges as a guide, the Philippines looks forward to aligning with others to advance the future of NI.

Key challenges are positioning NI as a specialty course in the Master's or PhD program; providing a regular NI position in the clinical setting; strengthening and positioning NI through issuances of policies and guidelines from the Department of Health; identifying the key roles and responsibilities of the nurse informaticists; building faculty teaching NI capacity; providing funding for NI studies on nursing improvement; and continuing to conduct nursing and health-related informatics initiatives.

Despite the challenges, these are promising perspectives to look welcome to advance the future of NI in the Philippines over the next decade. To have NI specialty programs, roles and responsibilities in the hospital and community are in place to support clinical learning. To that end, there will be more Filipino NI studies published in the top-tier informatics journals. And finally, Filipino nursing is committed to strengthen and sustain established networks and explore more partnerships within NI organizations worldwide.

References

Ambinder, E. P. (2005). Electronic health records. *Journal of Oncology Practice*, 1, pp.57–63. https://doi.org/10.1200/JOP.2005.1.2.57

Asian eHealth Information Network. (2011). *AeHIN history* [online]. Available at: https://www.asiaehealthinformationnetwork.org/ (Accessed 25 June 2021).

Barbosa, S. de F. F. (2017). Competencies related to informatics and information management for practicing nurses and nurses leaders in Brazil and South America. In IMIA, ed., *Forecasting informatics competencies for nurses in the future of connected health*, pp.77–85. https://doi.org/10.3233/978-1-61499-738-2-77

Barbosa, S. de F. F., Abbott, P., & Dal Sasso, G. T. M. (2021). Nursing in the digital health era. *Journal of Nursing Scholarship*, 53(1), pp.5–6. https://doi.org/10.1111/jnu.12620

Bernal, A. B., Tolentino, P. A., Gavino, A. I., Fontelo, P., Marcelo, A. B. Nursing informatics: Challenges to Philippine nursing curriculum. In AMIA Annual Symposium Proceedings, 2008 Nov 6, p.876 [online]. Available at: https://pubmed.ncbi.nlm.nih.gov/18998935/. (Accessed 5 July 2021).

Brasil. (2016). *Política nacional de informação e informática em saúde*.

Brasil. (2018a). *Brazil's 4th national action plan* [online]. Available at: https://www.opengovpartnership.org/wp-content/uploads/2020/08/Brazil_Action-Plan_2018-2021_Cycle-Update_EN.pdf (Accessed 5 July 2021).

Brasil. (2018b). *LEI Nº 13.709, DE 14 DE AGOSTO DE 2018* [online]. Available at: http://www.planalto.gov.br/ccivil_03/_ato2015-2018/2018/lei/L13709.htm (Accessed 5 July 2021).

Brasil. (2020). *Estratégia de Saúde Digital para o Brasil 2020–2028* (E. MS/CGD (ed.). 1st ed. [online]. http://bvsms.saude.gov.br/bvs/publicacoes/estrategia_saude_digital_Brasil.pdf (Accessed 5 July 2021).

Brasil. (2021). GO FAIR Brazil Office [online]. Available at: https://www.go-fair.org/go-fair-initiative/go-fair-offices/go-fair-brazil-office/ (Accessed 5 July 2021).

Caetano, R., Silva, A. B., Guedes, A. C. C. M., de Paiva, C. C. N., da Rocha Ribeiro, G., Santos, D. L., & da Silva, R. M. (2020). Challenges and opportunities for telehealth during the COVID-19 pandemic: Ideas on spaces and initiatives in the Brazilian context. *Cadernos de Saude Publica*, 36(5), pp.1–16. https://doi.org/10.1590/0102-311X00088920

Clara, M. C. S, Queiroz, A. C., Fonseca, M. P., Silva, M. P., & Andrade, L. D. F. (2020). Nursing management practices in health service. *SALUSVITA*, 39(2), pp.565–581.

CNAI – HIMMS | Gruppo Italiano Nursing Informatics (2021). [Online]. Available at: https://www.cnai.pro/post/cnai-himms (Accessed 23 July 23 2021).

Commission on Higher Education Memorandum Order 14 [online]. (2009). Available at: https://ched.gov.ph/wp-content/uploads/2017/10/CMO-No.14-s2009.pdf. (Accessed 25 June 2021).

Commission on Higher Education Memorandum Order 15 [online]. (2017). Available at: https://ched.gov.ph/wp-content/uploads/2017/10/CMO-15-s-2017.pdf (Accessed 25 June 2021).

Conselho Federal de Enfermagem - Brasil (n). Available at: http://www.cofen.gov.br/ (Accessed 26 December 2021).

Costi, L. R., Iwamoto, H. M., Neves, D. C. de O., & Caldas, C. A. M. (2017). Mortality from systemic erythematosus lupus in Brazil: Evaluation of causes according to the government health database. *Revista Brasileira de Reumatologia (English Edition)*, 57(6), pp.574–582. https://doi.org/10.1016/j.rbre.2017.09.001

D'Agostino, F. (2014). *Development of a nursing information system using stan-dard nursing language for creation of a nursing minimum data set.* Rome: Tor Vergata University.

D'Agostino, F., Sanson, G., Cocchieri, A., Vellone, E., Welton, J., Maurici, M., Alvaro, R., & Zega, M. (2017). Prevalence of nursing diagnoses as a measure of nursing complexity in a hospital setting. *Journal of Advanced Nursing*, 73(9), pp.2129–2142. https://doi.org/10.1111/jan.13285

D'Agostino, F., Vellone, E., Cocchieri, A., Welton, J., Maurici, M., Polistena, B., Spandonaro, F., Zega, M., Alvaro, R., & Sanson, G. (2019a) Nursing diagnoses as predictors of hospital length of stay: A prospective observational study. *Journal of Nursing Scholarship*, 51(1), pp.96–105. https://doi.org/10.1111/jnu.12444

D'Agostino, F., Vellone, E., Tontini, F., Zega, M., & Alvaro, R. (2012). Development of a computerized system using standard nursing language for creation of a nursing minimum data set. *Professioni Infermieristiche*, 65(2), pp.103–109.

D'Agostino, F., Zeffiro, V., Cocchieri, A., Vanalli, M., Ausili, D., Vellone, E., Zega, M., & Alvaro, R. (2019b). Impact of an electronic nursing documentation system on the nursing process accuracy. In Di Mascio, T. et al. (ed.), Methodologies and Intelligent Systems for Technology Enhanced Learning, 8th International Conference. MIS4TEL 2018. Advances in Intelligent Systems and Computing, Salamanca, Spain, vol 804. Cham: Springer, pp.247–252. https://doi.org/10.1007/978-3-319-98872-6_29

D'Agostino, F., Zega, M., Rocco, G., Luzzi, L., Vellone, E., & Alvaro, R. (2013). Impact of a nursing information system in clinical practice: A longitudinal study project. *Annali di Igiene: Medicina Preventiva e di Comunità*, 25(4), pp.329–341. https://doi.org/10.7416/ai.2013.1935

De Oliveira, N. B., & Peres, H. H. C. (2021). Quality of the documentation of the nursing process in clinical decision support systems. *Revista Latino-Americana de Enfermagem*, 29, p.e3426 [online]. https://doi.org/10.1590/1518-8345.4510.3426 (Accessed 5 July 2021).

Department of Health & Department of Science and Technology. (2014). *Philippines Ehealth strategic framework and plan, 2014–2020* [online]. Available at: http://ehealth.doh.gov.ph/index.php/transparency/overview#openModal11 (Accessed 25 June 2020).

e-HATID [online]. Available at: http://ehatid.ehealth.ph/ (Accessed 21 June 2021).

Gomes, P. de A. R., Farah, B. F., Rocha, R. S., Friedrich, D. B. de C., & Dutra, H. S. (2019). Electronic citizen record: An instrument for nursing care/Prontuário Eletrônico do Cidadão: Instrumento Para o Cuidado de Enfermagem. *Revista de Pesquisa Cuidado é Fundamental Online*, 11(5), pp.1226–1235. https://doi.org/10.9789/2175-5361.2019.v11i5.1226-1235

Grasiely, S., Albuquerque, E. De, Ribeiro, S., Costa, T., Amorim, H., Lúcia, A., Cabral, D. M., Serpa, P., & Batista, D. S. (2020). *Estratégia e-SUS atenção básica : dificuldades e perspectivas*, pp.399–405.

HCPA. (2020). *Sistema AGHUse*. Hospital de Clínicas de Porto Alegre [online]. Available at: https://www.hcpa.edu.br/institucional/tecnologia-da-informacao-e-comunicacao/institucional-sistema-aghuse (Accessed 27 July 2021).

Hermida, P. M. V. (2010). Desvelandoa implementação da sistematização da assistência de enfermagem. *Revista Brasileira de Enfermagem*, 57(6), pp.733–737. https://doi.org/10.1590/s0034-71672004000600021

IBGE. (2021). Instituto Brasileiro de Geografia e Estatística [online]. Available at: https://www.ibge.gov.br/ (Accessed 5 July 2021).

Informatics Nurses Society of the Philippines [online]. Available at: https://jrotoni.github.io/b3nc-rotoni-jeremy/csp1/index.html (Accessed 21 July 2021).

Italian ICNP Research & Development Centre. (2021). [online]. Available at: https://www.icn.ch/what-we-do/projects/ehealth/about-icnp/icn-accredited-centres-icnpr-research-development/italian (Accessed 22 July 2021).

Kharrat, F. G. Z., Miyoshi, N. S. B., Cobre, J., de Azevedo-Marques, J. M., de Azevedo-Marques, P. M., & Botazzo Delbem, A. C. (2020). Feature sensitivity criterion-based sampling strategy from the Optimization based on Phylogram Analysis (Fs-OPA) and Cox regression applied to mental disorder datasets. *PLoS ONE*, 15(7), pp.1–25. https://doi.org/10.1371/journal.pone.0235147

Lacerda, T. C., Hammes, J. F., Fantonelli, M., Monguilhott, E., & Wazlawick, R. S. (2020). e-SUS APS strategy : Case of success on Primary Care informatization in Brazil. *Journal of Health Informatics*, 12(4), pp.138–143.

Liaskos, J., & Mantas, J. (2002). Nursing information system. *Studies in Health Technology and Informatics*, 65, pp.258–265.

Locsin, R., & Purnell, M. (2015). Advancing the theory of technological competency as caring in nursing: The universal technological domain. *International Journal for Human Caring* [online], 19(2), pp.50–54. Available at: https://humancaring.org/resources/Online%20Presentations/2021/Advancing%20TCCN%20UTD.pdf. (Accessed 5 July 2021).

Lytle, K. S., Westra, B. L., Whittenburg, L., Adams, M., Akre, M., Ali, S., Furukawa, M., Hartleben, S., Hook, M., Johnson, S. G., Settergren, T. T., & Thibodeaux, M. (2021). Information models offer value to standardize electronic health record flowsheet data: A fall prevention exemplar. *Journal of Nursing Scholarship*, 53(3), pp.306–314. https://doi.org/10.1111/jnu.12646

Mahrenbach, L. C., Mayer, K., & Pfeffer, J. (2018). Policy visions of big data: Views from the Global South. *Third World Quarterly*, 39(10), pp.1861–1882. https://doi.org/10.1080/01436597.2018.1509700

Mazzoleni, B., Ausili, D., Gagliano, C., Genovese, C., Santin, C., & Rigon, L. A. (2018). Standardized nursing terminologies in nursing education and clinical practice: An Italian survey. *L'Infermiere*, 55(1), pp.E18–32.

Meirelles, R. F., & Cunha, F. J. A. P. (2020). Autenticidade e preservação de Registros Eletrônicos em Saúde: proposta de modelagem da cadeia de custódia das informações orgânicas do Sistema Único de Saúde. *Revista Eletrônica de Comunicação, Informação e Inovação Em Saúde*, 14(3), pp.580–596. https://doi.org/10.29397/reciis.v14i3.2117

Ministério da Educação. (2020). *Empresas brasileiras de serviços hospitalares* [online]. Available at: https://www.gov.br/ebserh/pt-br/hospitais-universitarios/regiao-nordeste/hu-ufma/governanca/superintendencia/aghu (Accessed 23 July 2021).

Nabinger Menna Barreto, L., Barragan da Silva, M., Tsuma Gaedke Nomura, A., de Fátima Lucena, A., & de Abreu Almeida, M. (2020). Clinical evolution of nursing outcome indicators in patients with ineffective breathing pattern. *Revista Eletronica de Enfermagem*, 22, pp.1–8.

National Institute of Health [online]. Available at: https://nih.upm.edu.ph/institute/national-telehealth-center. (Accessed 5 July 2021).

National Telehealth Center [online]. Available at: https://telehealth.ph/history/. (Accessed 5 July 2021).

Nomura, A. T. G., Almeida, M.de A., & Pruinelli, L. (2021). *Information model on pain management: An analysis of big data.* https://doi.org/10.1111/jnu.12638

Nomura, A. T. G., Almeida, M.de A., Johnson, S., & Pruinelli, L. (2021). *Pain information model and its potential for predictive analytics: Applicability of a big data science framework*, pp.315–322. https://doi.org/10.1111/jnu.12648

Nomura, A. T. G., Pruinelli, L., Da Silva, M. B., Lucena, A. D. F., & Almeida, M. D. A. (2018). Quality of electronic nursing records: The impact of educational interventions during a hospital accreditation process. *CIN: Computers Informatics Nursing*, 36(3), pp.127–132. https://doi.org/10.1097/CIN.0000000000000390

Paese, F., Sasso, G. T. M. D., & Colla, G. W. (2018). Structuring methodology of the computerized nursing process in emergency care units. *Revista Brasileira de Enfermagem*, 71(3), pp.1079–1084. https://doi.org/10.1590/0034-7167-2016-0619

Park, H. A., Min, Y. H., Kim, Y., Lee, M. K., & Lee, Y. (2011). Development of detailed clinical models for nursing assessments and nursing interventions. *Healthcare Informatics Research*, 17(4), pp.244–252. https://doi.org/10.4258/hir.2011.17.4.244

Philippine Council of Health Research and Development (PCHRD) (online). Available at: https://www.pchrd.dost.gov.ph/programs-and-services/create-article/6556-community-health-information-tracking-system-chits (Accessed 5 July 6 2021).

Pires, A. U. B., Lucena, A.de F., Behenck, A., & Heldt, E. (2020). Results of the nursing outcomes classification/NOC for patients with obsessive-compulsive disorder. *Revista Brasileira de Enfermagem*, 73(1), p.e20180209. https://doi.org/10.1590/0034-7167-2018-0209

Rabelo-Silva, E. R., Cavalcanti, A.C.D., Caldas, M.C.R.G., Lucena, A.d.F., Almeida, M.d.A., Linch, G.F.D.C., da Silva, M.B., & Müller-Staub, M. (2017). Advanced nursing process quality: Comparing the International Classification for Nursing Practice (ICNP) with the NANDA-International (NANDA-I) and Nursing Interventions Classification (NIC). *Journal of Clinical Nursing*, 26(3–4), pp.379–387. https://doi.org/10.1111/jocn.13387. Blackwell Publishing Ltd.

RxBox [online]. Available at: https://rxbox.chits.ph/what_is_rxbox/. (Accessed 21 June 2021).

Sanni Ali, M., Ichihara, M. Y., Lopes, L. C., Barbosa, G. C. G., Pita, R., Carreiro, R. P., Dos Santos, D. B., Ramos, D., Bispo, N., Raynal, F., Canuto, V., De Araujo Almeida, B., Fiaccone, R. L., Barreto, M. E., Smeeth, L., & Barreto, M. L. (2019).

Administrative data linkage in Brazil: Potentials for health technology assessment. *Frontiers in Pharmacology*, 10(Sep), pp.1–20. https://doi.org/10.3389/fphar.2019.00984

Sanson, G., Alvaro, R., Cocchieri, A., Vellone, E., Welton, J., Maurici, M., Zega, M., & D'Agostino, F. (2019a) Nursing diagnoses, interventions and activities as described by a nursing minimum data set: A prospective study in an oncology hospital setting. *Cancer Nursing*, 42(2), pp.E39–47. https://doi.org/10.1097/NCC.0000000000000581

Sanson, G., Vellone, E., Kangasniemi, M., Alvaro, R., & D'Agostino F. (2017). Impact of nursing diagnoses on patient and organisational outcomes: A systematic literature review. *Journal of Clinical Nursing*, 26(23–24), pp.3764–3783. https://doi.org/10.1111/jocn.13717

Sanson, G., Welton, J., Vellone, E., Cocchieri, A., Maurici, M., Zega, M., Alvaro, R. and D'Agostino, F. (2019b) Enhancing the performance of predictive models for hospital mortality by adding nursing data. *International Journal of Medical Informatics*, 125, pp.79–85. https://doi.org/10.1016/j.ijmedinf.2019.02.009

Savini, S., Iovino, P., Monaco, D., Marchini, R., Di Giovanni, T., Donato, G., Pulimeno, A., Matera, C., Quintavalle, G., & Turci, C. (2021). A family nurse-led intervention for reducing health services' utilization in individuals with chronic diseases: The ADVICE pilot study. *International Journal of Nursing Sciences*, In press. https://doi.org/10.1016/j.ijnss.2021.05.001

Silva, A. B., da Silva, R. M., Ribeiro, G. R., Guedes, A. C. C. M., Santos, D. L., Nepomuceno, C. C., & Caetano, R. (2020). Three decades of telemedicine in Brazil: Mapping the regulatory framework from 1990 to 2018. *PLoS ONE*, 15(11 November), pp.1–21. https://doi.org/10.1371/journal.pone.0242869

Stelmach, R., & Cruz, Á. A. (2017). *The Paradox of Asthma: Neglect, Burden, and Big Data*, 43(3), pp.159–160.

Sumabat, K. R. (2010). *History of nursing informatics in the Philippines* [online]. Available at: ng_informatics.pdf. (Accessed 5 July 2021).

Venkatesh, V., Morris, M. G., Davis, G. B., & Davis, F. D. (2003). User acceptance of information technology: Toward a unified view. *MIS Quarterly*, 27(3), pp.425–478.

Werley, H. H., Devine, E. C., Zorn, C. R., Ryan, P., & Westra, B. L. (1991). The nursing minimum data set: Abstraction tool for standardized, comparable, essential data. *American Journal of Public Health*, 81(4), pp.421–426. https://doi.org/10.2105/ajph.81.4.421

Wireless Access for Health [online]. Available at: https://wah.ph/#/auth. (Accessed 23 June 2021).

World Health Organization [online]. (2010). Available at: https://www.who.int/pmnch/events/partners_forum/ICT_transforming_Healthcare_Education_Philippines.pdf. (Accessed 5 July 2021).

Zeffiro, V., Sanson, G., Carboni, L., Malatesta, A., Vellone, E., Alvaro, R., & D'Agostino, F. (2018). The nursing-led in-patient unit: A descriptive study of nursing care delivered. *Igiene e Sanità Pubblica*, 74(4), pp.359–376.

Zeffiro, V., Sanson, G., Welton, J., Maurici, M., Malatesta, A., Carboni, L., Vellone, E., Alvaro, R., & D'Agostino, F. (2020). Predictive factors of a prolonged length of stay in a community nursing-led unit: A retrospective cohort study. *Journal of Clinical Nursing*, 29(23–24), pp.4685–4696. https://doi.org/10.1111/jocn.15509

Zega, M., D'Agostino, F., Bowles, K. H., De Marinis, M. G., Rocco, G., Vellone, E., & Alvaro, R. (2014). Development and validation of a computerized assessment form to support nursing diagnosis. *International Journal of Nursing Knowledge*, 25(1), pp.22–29. https://doi.org/10.1111/2047-3095.12008

Zega, M., French, S., Vicario, G., Vellone, E., & Alvaro, R. (2010). The chronic patient and the nurse-managed hospital unit. *Igiene e Sanità Pubblica*, 66(4), pp.551–562.

Chapter 10

South Africa's Healthcare Systems, Technology and Nursing

Graham Wright, Helen J. Betts,
Chrispin Kabuya and Henry Adams

Contents

DOI: 10.4324/9781003054849-10

Introduction

The continent of Africa is huge at 30.37 million square kilometres. It is large enough to accommodate the United States of America, China, India, Japan, Mexico and many European countries with 20.4% of the world's landmass. South Africa, at 1,219,090 km², is almost twice the size of the state of Texas. The Indian Ocean borders the east coast, and the Atlantic Ocean borders the west allocating South Africa a coastline totalling 2,798 km. The country has 11 official languages with the government using English for communications; however, only 8.4% of the population have English as their first language. The nine regional provinces each have a distinct character. South Africa can be described as both a developed and under-developed country. The World Bank classifies it as an upper-middle-income country with a population of 59,309,635 of which 54% live below the poverty line. Corrado Gini, the Italian statistician and sociologist developed the Gini Coefficient or *GINI Index* which demonstrates the income/wealth inequality within societies. The GINI Index for South Africa shows the gap of 0.63 between rich and poor as the highest in the world.

Many authors, including those of this chapter, have cautioned about compelling nurses to collect data that has no practical use for them, in other words, 'bean counting for some report' (O'Mahony & Wright, 2014). With all digital enablement, the key is to capture information generated directly from the work being done. In a clinical setting, most events happen between a healthcare professional, a nurse or an administrator and the patient. Presently, nurses do not have ownership of data collection and data use for nursing care. In the public sector, they function in ways more akin to nursing in the 1960s in Europe and the 1980s in the former Soviet countries, in that nurses do everything that doctors do not have time or want to do. In the more technically advanced regions of the world, professions allied to medicine took over many of these functional tasks and made them their own professions, for example, physiotherapists and occupational therapists. In South Africa almost every day, on average, 60 people are murdered, 40 people are killed in road traffic accidents and 190 people die of AIDS-related illnesses. This description paints a picture with which to understand the current nursing in South Africa.

Technology and the General Population— Understanding Nursing in South Africa

To grasp the role of nurses in Africa today, one must first 'see' the context within which they work. The majority of Africa is rural with a vastly different way of life compared to Europe or North America. Most of the populace has never used a computer and many have never seen one. In 2013, only about 45% of the urban population had electricity and an estimated 19% of the population had access to electricity in rural Sub-Saharan Africa (Wright, 2013). The Internet World Statistics for Africa, 2016, shows that only 9.3% of people across the African continent were Internet users. In contrast, mobile phone ownership is growing in African regions with mobile phone use and Internet access successfully sidestepping the era of desktop computers and landlines (Wright, 2018). South Africa has, like other African countries, leap-frogged the computer age with mobile phones. However, most people cannot afford data for use on their phones to use any apps. An estimated 92 million handsets are owned by a population of just under 60 million.

The Burden of Disease

South Africa has a high burden of disease, which can be seen in Table 10.1 showing the incidence of HIV/AIDS across countries in Southern Africa.

The Central Intelligence Agency (CIA) World Factbook compares the percentage of adults (aged 15-49) living with HIV/AIDS across the seven countries (Central Intelligence Agency, 2011). Lesotho is a landlocked nation surrounded by South Africa whilst six other countries form its borders; and together, these countries present a solid block of the highest incidence of HIV/AIDS in the world. In 2019, UNAIDS estimated that 38 million people were living with HIV worldwide, with the World Health Organisation (WHO) stating that 70% of the disease burden is situated in Sub-Saharan Africa (UNAIDS, 2020; WHO, 2021b). South Africa is also experiencing an extraordinary tuberculosis (TB) epidemic which can partly be attributed to HIV/AIDS, as people are more susceptible to TB when their immune system is weakened by HIV (Singh et al., 2007). Amongst the 22 high-burden TB countries, cited by the WHO in 2009, 73% of TB cases in South Africa also had HIV (WHO, 2009). The UNAIDS Report indicates that South Africa had approximately 200,000 new HIV infections in 2019, with women having the

Table 10.1 Seven Southern Africa Countries with the Percentage of HIV/AIDS Population

Eswatini	Lesotho	Botswana	South Africa	Zimbabwe	Namibia	Mozambique
27.10	23.10	22.20	17.30	13.40	12.70	12.10

highest number of new cases at 120,000. However, this is a drop in the new infection incidence in all age ranges and genders with a total HIV incidence per 1,000 population of 3.98. In 2010 and 2015 the incidence was 9.48 and 5.94 respectively. In 2019, 72,000 people of all ages died of AIDS-related illnesses in South Africa. This is a 61% decline since 2010. There were also 7,500,000 people living with HIV, of whom 4,700,000 were women over the age of 15 years in South Africa. The number of women living with HIV has increased from 3,600,000 in 2010. Adolescent girls and young women in Sub-Saharan Africa account for one in four infections. The overall number of people living with HIV has risen even though the AIDS-related death rate and new HIV infection rate have declined. This suggests that those of the population who have treatment are responding to it. However, South Africa has not achieved the testing and treatment target set by UNAIDS for antiretroviral therapy coverage of 81% of the HIV infected population by 2020.

South Africa has two distinct health services: the private healthcare system, servicing 9 million people and the public sector, serving almost 50 million people. Table 10.2 shows the estimated number of clinics and hospitals for the private and public healthcare systems. The total Gross Domestic Product (GDP) spent in each of these sectors is very similar, reflecting the disproportionate distribution of resources between the private and public systems (Maphumulo & Bhengu, 2019).

Nurse's Role and Training

The South African Qualifications Authority (SAQA, 2021) is 'responsible for the recognition of professional bodies and registration of professional designations.' Nurse education in South Africa is governed by the Nursing Council with validated programmes approved for Certificate, Diploma and Degree level registration implemented in 2015. The range of postgraduate diplomas approved by the Council includes the main Nursing specialities together with Health Services Management and Nursing Education. The government

Table 10.2 Estimated Number of Clinics and Hospitals in South Africa in 2021 Calculated by the Authors from Various Audits and Public Lists (Ndlovu et al., 2020)

Public Clinics	Public Hospitals	Private Clinics	Private Hospitals
3,869	422	610	203

funding of these specialities relates to the lack of medical doctors in rural areas. Another government initiative is the contractual agreement with all funded nurses and doctors that they spend a year, post qualification, in a rural setting. Some private hospitals are licensed to train nurses and all three major, private hospital groups have nurse training colleges. There are also several private, nurse training colleges at the diploma level, while the degree-granting programmes are university-based in Departments of Nursing.

Additionally, some universities use online learning management systems, such as Moodle and Blackboard; however, the expensive data costs put them beyond the access of most students (Wright et al., 2017). The onset of COVID-19 spearheaded the use of information technology in all South Africa's education sectors, including video conferencing, Webinar and online tuition of programmes, which was enabled by the government supplying free data to both staff and students. Changing staff and student behaviour, as well as reducing the costs of online education has allowed most Higher Education programmes to continue throughout the COVID lockdowns.

Healthcare System, Technologies Used and Nursing

South Africa's private healthcare in the major towns and cities is like the rest of the developed world, including acute, clinic, specialist and general practitioners. However, this healthcare is only available at high and rapidly increasing price levels. As an example, a family of two adults pay around 6,700 Rand (490 US dollars) a month for a mid-range health scheme which is approximately twice the monthly minimum wage. The old person's grant for those over the age of 60 years is 1,890 Rand or 128$ a month. All healthcare professionals in the South African private healthcare market, except nurses, are self-employed, e.g., physicians, physiotherapists.

In general, the private hospitals and clinics collect data for billing purposes, staff record work undertaken and limitation of exposure to legal liability i.e., billable hours, hours worked, complaints registers. Nurses spend an inordinate amount of their time on manual recording, collating and entering data from which they receive no information pertinent to nursing care.

The public healthcare system can employ healthcare IT professionals, within its responsibilities. In public hospitals, there is limited use of information systems and no consistency of systems either within or across the nine provinces, for example:

1. IALCH (Inkosi Albert Luthuli Central Hospital) is an academic, referral-based hospital situated in Durban. It is owned by the Provincial Kwa Zulu Natal (KZN) Department of Health (DoH) and managed through a Public-Private Partnership (PPP). It was opened in 2002 and has 846 beds, including 46 Burns Unit beds, 75 Intensive Care Unit beds and 96 High-Care beds and a capacity for 200 additional beds. The hospital has 16 operating theatres, two trauma operating theatres and one burns operating theatre (Aramesh, 2019). IALCH has a fully, digitally enabled, paperless Electronic Patient Record (EPR) IT system covering all aspects of care, including a Patient Administration and Clinical Information System. The system also has integrated with the Radiology Information System and has an interface to the pathology service provider, the National Health Laboratory Service (NHLS). Data warehousing and data analytics are also available.

2. The Western Cape Province (WC) has a well-established Patient Administration System (PAS) and Master Patient Index (MPI). It is the only province with a functioning provincial MPI with a few satellite applications such as Discharge Summaries.

None of the other eight provinces has a provincial-wide MPI, which is a fundamental building block on top of which electronic medical record (EMR) applications can run and support improvements in health outcomes.

In rural areas, healthcare provision in the public sector is provided by district and sub-district hospitals, community health centres (CHCs), clinics and in some cases, mobile clinics. It is within these constraints that applications to support nursing need to be considered.

Private Healthcare Systems

The provision of acute and ambulatory care in the private healthcare sector is mostly dominated by three main private hospital groups, namely Netcare, MediClinic and Life hospital system groups. Services provided include private laboratories, X-ray, specialists, General Practitioners (GP), physiotherapy and psychology which are all independent businesses. Pathology and radiology services are provided by private specialists who form administrative companies/trusts to administer their businesses. Pathology is dominated by three private organisations: Ampath, Lancet and Pathcare laboratory services that undertake over 90% of all pathology performed in the private market.

The legislation restricts these privately owned companies from offering services in the public sector, which is the domain of the NHLS that equally may not operate in the private market. Radiology services have a similar divided structure with private associations/groups/trusts operating in this domain.

The hospital group simply provides an environment in which healthcare professionals can deliver their services. The hospital group provides the beds, nurses, theatres, food, security and patient administration and billing systems. However, they do not undertake the administration and billing for the healthcare professionals that make use of their facilities.

The challenge this presents to digital transformation is that applications are not designed around the patient, which is a prerequisite to support digital enablement for such functions as nursing. The patient is not the hospital's customer: The customer is the physician. There is neither a financial incentive nor a legislative imperative to ensure the implementation of patient-centric applications that focus on improving patient care and outcomes. The same scenario afflicts general practitioners who have no legislative or commercial imperative to use EMR applications. Applications are geared towards checking the patient's ability to pay and then billing the patient or insurer.

Public Healthcare Systems

Each province is responsible for the management and staffing of its hospitals and clinics. Seven of the nine provinces have an academic, public hospital with an associated medical school. These provincial, academic medical systems are often regarded as centres of excellence. Mpumalanga and Northern Cape are the two historical exceptions because they are situated in the previously disadvantaged universities of independent black communities in the apartheid era. A province's healthcare services include district and sub-district hospitals that operate on a 24-hour basis; community healthcare centres that have a few acute care beds; and clinics that operate limited, usually daytime hours. The hospitals are the primary care providers and are staffed by emergency and primary care physicians. The departments of a district hospital include Emergency, Maternity, TB, Medical, and General Surgery, which create a training environment for GPs. In 2017, there were more than 20 million nurses worldwide, with over four million in the United States of America. The number of nurses and midwives per 10,000 population is 216.70 in Sweden, 145.5 per in the United States of America, but only 13.1 in South Africa (WHO, 2021a).

Although the principles of the nursing process are taught during nurse training, it is not used in practice. The nurses only have time for the urgent and important aspects of patient care due to the vast numbers of patients attending clinics or hospitals (Wright et al., 2014a). People attending CHCs, Rural Clinics and Mobile Clinics in rural South Africa, such as in the Eastern Cape, often walk long distances (10–20 km) and then wait all day to see a nurse and sometimes overnight. Many clinics have neither water nor electricity and often run short of essential supplies that are delivered by a four-wheeled, drive vehicle. There are no public ambulances in these areas for clinic use.

Information Collected in Clinics

The District Health Information System (DHIS) is used in South Africa, within the government's District Health Management Information System (DHMIS) programme for collecting aggregated data from health facilities. DHMIS includes 'the people; policies, procedures; hardware; software; networks and datasets required to ensure a well-functioning information system' (National Department of Health, 2011). Three Interlinked Electronic Registers (TIER) is a system for entering manually collected information on disease entities for public health purposes. It is 'a 3-tier approach to monitoring that includes a paper-based system making up tier 1, an electronic version of the paper register as the middle tier or tier 2, and full electronic medical record software at the 3rd tier' (Osler & Boulle, 2010). In 2010, the Department of Health announced the move of HIV and Anti Retro Viral (ARV) therapy monitoring into TIER.Net. Since the introduction of TIER, nurses send paper-based data to data capturers who enter it into spreadsheets to produce data register reports for the Department of Health, which had a target of 10,000 data capturers working in CHCs and clinics. TIER is still the method of data collection in 2021 with separate COVID-19 data collection systems for the WHO and DHIS (Osler & Boulle, 2010).

Information Capture in Clinics

As described above, the bulk of primary healthcare (PHC) in South Africa is provided by nurses at CHCs and clinics in the public health sector. Data at CHCs and clinics are handwritten in registers by nurses predominantly for Monitoring and Evaluation (M+E). Nurses or data capturers create the monthly summary report by calculating the number of events in each disease register. The report is submitted to the District Health Information System 2 (DHIS2). This monthly summary report includes the numbers of administered immunisations, sputum samples collected for tuberculosis testing, the number of persons diagnosed with tuberculosis, and laboratory results for human immunodeficiency virus (HIV) positive patients. Nurses also write the care management on paper sheets and cards which are retained by the patient.

A study (Odama, 2010) in the OR Tambo District of the Eastern Cape showed that there were major issues with data quality due to the staff's high workload. Most of the care in clinics was provided by nurses, mainly without medical oversight, using government flow charts and protocols that the nurses initiated and implemented. Often, nurses worked all day seeing one patient every ten minutes during which time they were required to assess and treat the patient and write in the register. Only one copy of each register in the clinic is concerned with a specific disorder i.e., HIV, TB, Diabetes or Antenatal Care. Some clinics reported having over 20 such registers. The nurses did not have time to hunt for the required register. If it was not in the treatment room in which the nurse was seeing the patient, then the nurse would plan to write it later. Patients who come with multiple pathologies can only be recorded in one register with a single reason for attending. However, the patient-held record should note more than one reason for attendance. Clinic nurses reported that many patients forget or lose their patient-held record, so a new record is started at successive clinic visits, often in a child's school notebook rather than an official health record card.

Several studies (Wright & Odama, 2012; Odama et al., 2014a, b) showed that there were major gaps in the data collected for planning and programme management. Odama highlighted that around 40% of patients attending clinics were not recorded and in addition, the counts in the registers did not match the monthly summary reports submitted to the District Health Authority. Additionally, nurses work under conditions of supply/medicine shortages. In a national audit (Department of Health, 2013), clinics reported a 54% availability of medicines and supplies and a shortage of ARV drugs. In these district clinics, most nurses are overwhelmed by the daily onslaught of too many patients, against a backdrop of many clerical functions, lack of materials and equipment, lengthy power outages and surrounded by abject poverty.

Technology Adoption in Rural Clinics

Starting in 2009, the Walter Sisulu University Health Informatics Research Team conducted a series of studies beginning with a proof-of-concept study on technology adoption at the clinic level. The researchers found that nurses in rural clinics rejected the use of computers but were comfortable using mobile devices as the majority owned and used a mobile phone. Most clinic nurses had never used or seen a fixed device such as a desktop computer; whereas they readily adopted the mobile tablet device, as it resembled a mobile phone in function. Two android Elite 9.7-inch tablets were purchased and configured by the team and the data collection forms were designed by replicating the paper forms of the paper-based tuberculosis screening tool routinely used in PHC (O'Mahony & Wright, 2014).

Final Project–Part 1: Building an Information System

Following the proof-of-concept study, the Sisulu research team chose the Mthakulo Community Health Centre (CHC), about 30 minutes travel from Mthatha, as the site for an in-depth, nursing data capture study alongside a time and motion (T&M) study. It is a rural CHC serving around 100,000 people who live in relative poverty. The team observed how routine data were generated, stored and used at the CHC before designing the data flow. Routine data were recorded in several clinic registers across various consultation rooms. The registers included the Isoniazid Preventive Therapy (IPT) Register, Chronic Diseases Management Register, HIV Counselling and Testing Register, Chronic Disease and Minor Ailments Register (Tick register) and the TB Register. Data from the registers was separated into clinical data that were coded into XForms, and demographic data that were coded as HTML5 forms to be used in the MPI application. A detailed description of the methodology and technical specifications for this study can be found in (Kabuya et al., 2014).

The benefits realised from the use of tablet computers included both personal and operational benefits for the nurses and the patients. Saving time and the reduction of recording errors were major benefits. Nurses did not spend time writing in registers either when the patient was with them or at the end of the day or week. This enabled the nurses to have improved communication with individual patients within a single consultation and indeed enabled patients either to have more time with a nurse or nurses to see more patients within the working day. Nurses had improved access to statistics and patient data during consultations giving them more confidence that their care would be of direct benefit to the patient.

The construction of the monthly reports became easier and less time-consuming because nurses did not have to re-enter the recorded data manually into a computer. Improved data quality, reliability and quick access to summary and aggregate routine data not only enhanced the clinic experience for nurses and patients but also meant that reporting to the district level became easier and less burdensome. No calculations were required by the nurses to produce more accurate monthly reports. The technical design of the forms on the tablet computers enabled standard reporting from the data stored in the SQL database and further analysis, exporting and reporting were possible such as to the Department of Health's TIER system to capture anonymised data for government statistics and reports to WHO and funding bodies such as PEPFAR.

The patients had reduced waiting times and clerking patients into the clinic was quicker as there was instant retrieval of each patient's demographic details and clinic number from the MPI system. The patients could be reassured that the nurse caring for them had more reliable information about their medical issues which would lead to better prescribed care.

The use of tablet computers by the nurses for this data collection was unique and improved data quality and influenced the development of apps for DHIS2 and similar databases. The study detail can be found in (Kabuya et al., 2014).

Final Project—Part 2: Time and Motion Study

The final project combined information gathered from the previous studies and included a 12-week nurses' workload and activity analysis. This T&M study covered six normal nursing behaviours before and after the introduction of tablet computers to collect patient data (Wright et al., 2014b). Phase One of the study was undertaken with the nurses using the registers in their normal work processes. In Phase Two, the nurses used tablet computers to collect patient data during the consultation. The T&M list of activities was based on recorded nurses' activity during consultations in a study by the team at another clinic (Wright et al., 2014b).

There was a shift in the time spent on activities within the two phases by not having to record all the patient demographic details. In Phase One some patients had 31 activities recorded whereas in Phase Two 23 activities were the maximum recorded. The research assistants commented that the nurses in Phase One tended to talk to the patient whilst undertaking activities and write in the registers between each activity thus giving the perception that the focus of the consultation was on writing in the registers. In Phase Two, the nurses captured the data on the tablet computers at the end of all activities or the consultation. This changed the nurses' behaviour from focusing on writing registers to conducting a patient-focused consultation hence improving patient care. Where there was minimal eye contact while writing in the registers, there was eye contact throughout the consultation between the nurse and the patient with the tablet devices. The analysis of the captured patient data collected on the tablet computers was complete and accurate.

Working Practices

While the research outlined above demonstrates the feasibility of what is possible with minimal technology investments in a rural clinic, the reality is somewhat different in both hospitals and clinics in the Eastern Cape. The Qaukeni Ingquza Hill sub-district in the Eastern Cape has 77.3% of its people living under the national poverty line; and 99% of the inhabitants are African whose commonly used language is isiXhosa. Qaukeni has two gateway clinics that refer patients to the two district hospitals, as part of 20 clinics, plus 2 Mobile clinics, serving a population of 303,379 (Ingquza Hill Local Municipality, 2020). In one of the clinics, all clinical data is recorded on paper by the nurses and processed by six clerks who file the paper records and enter the data. Three clerks are employed by the DoH and the other three by the Non-Governmental Organisation (NGO), TB/HIV Care.

The data clerks use a spreadsheet to collect data for Tier.net for HIV (basic information on CD4 counts, Viral Loads and drugs) and TB data recording. A simple standalone, Patient Medical Record System (PMRS) that runs on a SQL database is used to record basic identity data, cell number and the paper-file number. All other data, including laboratory data, are extracted from paper records, or looked up online on TrakCare (the NHLS results online reporting system) and entered manually into the patient paper-based clinical record. However, the nurses still complete the registers first.

Recent Developments in Digital Applications for Mobile Phones

1. MomConnect links over two million pregnant women and new mothers supporting and improving maternal and child health using free, cell phone technologies. The messages are available in all eleven official South African languages, which is unusual due to difficulties of translation (MomConnect—National Department of Health, 2020).
2. The COVID-19 pandemic heralded major behavioural changes in all populations particularly the collection of COVID-19 data at a personal level. The DHIS2 made available a COVID-19 module in April 2020 and this was rapidly installed on the DHIS2 system across Africa with the option of using mobile phones to collect data (Technical Guidance Publications, 2020).
3. The NHLS TrakCare pathology results server can be accessed via a cell phone with a web browser.

While these health applications for use on mobile smartphones demonstrate progress in health information technology in South Africa, it needs to be set in context. The official language of the government and its departments is English but only 11% of the population speak it fluently. The majority of the population have at least one mobile phone, although many of them are simple phones and therefore cannot utilise these digital developments. In addition, the cost of data is prohibitive for a sizable proportion of the population. Therefore, these digital applications have a limited number of potential users.

Conclusion

Most rural hospitals did not have patient records departments until recently with many patients still carrying their notes, written in school exercise books, which were often lost, with no backup notes kept at the clinic or hospital. In an endeavour to address these issues, the government introduced the National Health Insurance (NHI) scheme in each province as a two-year, pilot study starting in 2016. This effort to bring some of the private health facilities within the reach of those without private insurance has not yet shown results. Nothing appears to have changed and no actions seem to have commenced since the pilot sites results were reported. Indeed, one part-time GP observed that he seemed to be the only doctor working at any of the 20 clinics in the Qaukeni Ingquza Hill region.

The national standard certification process of Electronic Health Records (EHRs) (NDOH, 2014) and the 2008 government ban on the procurement of computerised patient systems was an attempt to bring together public and private sectors supported by the NHI scheme. The government has been made aware of the major difficulties in the data collection systems. 'In 2014, an estimated 3,000 out of 4,000 public sector clinics in South Africa were using TIER.Net in one of the three phases of implementation. As of 2017, TIER 3 was still in its pilot phase'(Etoori et al., 2020).

Etoori and colleagues (2020) explored the differences between the treatment and residency status of HIV patients between April 2014 and August 2017 in a rural South African setting by analysing the national treatment database (TIER.Net). These researchers found major data integrity issues including: misclassification of patient outcomes by 36%; and errors in Anti-Retroviral Treatment (ART) initiation reason, baseline CD4, health facility attended, Point-of-contact Interactive Record Linkage (PIRL), time since the last appointment, age, and ART refill schedule. Data held in the TIER.Net also underestimated mortality and overestimated the number of patients who had left the programme.

The COVID-19 pandemic has again illustrated the diversity of healthcare provision between the rich and poor countries in the world. Ownership and creation of wealth together with intellectual property rights and patents ensure that the wealthy countries obtain and control the manufacturing and distribution of vaccines. Maslow (1943) reminds us that the lack of basic physiological needs prevents attainment to higher levels such as when a mother puts her children to sleep on the floor of their wattle and daub hut, hungry and with little hope for a better future. African countries are considered 'Third World' or 'Underdeveloped' except for a few 'developing countries.' The lack of resources, both human and material, has been apparent in a multitude of papers and reports over the last decade. The west has taken raw materials out of African countries and not supported those countries in developing the transformation manufacturing processes of raw materials into added-value goods including mined diamonds and precious metals. The continent also supplies cheap labour in terms of call centres for companies that then do not deliver their products to African customers.

The health infrastructure and personnel need to change if we hope to achieve universal health coverage in Africa. Nurses have many roles in the absence of other healthcare professionals and particularly in the massive rural areas of low-density populations and difficult travelling terrain. Paradoxically the COVID-19 pandemic has forced Africa to develop new public healthcare data systems. Hence there is Nursing Informatics in Africa, but not as we know it.

Acknowledgements

We would like to recognise the contribution of the Walter Sisulu University Health Informatics Research Team, including Don O'Mahony, Parimalaranie Yogeswaran, Antony Odama, Rajeev Rao Eashwar, Frederick Govere and the late Malcolm Ellis.

References List

Aramesh, K. (2019). Situation analysis. In *Advancing global bioethics*. London: Springer, pp.21–42.

Central Intelligence Agency. (2011). *The world factbook: Countries/South Africa*.

Department of Health. (2013). *The national health care facilities baseline audit: National summary report*, pp.1–75.

Etoori, D., Wringe, A., Kabudula, C. W., Renju, J., Rice, B., Gomez-Olive, F. X., & Reniers, G. (2020). Misreporting of patient outcomes in the South African National HIV treatment database: Consequences for programme planning, monitoring, and evaluation. *Frontiers in Public Health*, 8(100), pp.1–21. https://doi.org/10.3389/fpubh.2020.00100. PMID: 32318534; PMCID: PMC7154050.

Ingquza Hill Local Municipality. (2020). *Integrated development plan 2019/20 Financial Year* [online]. Available at: https://www.cogta.gov.za/cgta_2016/wp-content/uploads/2020/11/INGQUZA-Hill-FINAL-IDP-2019-2020.pdf (Accessed 28 May 2021).

Kabuya, C., Wright, G., Odama, A., & O'Mahoney, D. (2014). Routine data for disease surveillance in the undeveloped region of the OR Tambo District of the Eastern Cape Province. In *Studies in health technology and informatics*. Amsterdam, the Netherlands: IOS Press, pp.103–107.

Maphumulo, W. T. & Bhengu, B. R. (2019). Challenges of quality improvement in the healthcare of South Africa post-apartheid: A critical review. *Curationis*, 42(1), pp.1–9. https://doi.org/10.4102/curationis.v42i1.1901.PMID: 31170800.

Maslow, A. (1943). A theory of human motivation. *Psychological Review*, 50, pp.370–396.

MomConnect – National Department of Health [online]. (2020). Available at: http://www.health.gov.za/momconnect/ (Accessed 28 May 2021).

National Department of Health. (2011). *District health management information system (DHIMS).*

Ndlovu, N., Day, C., Gray, A. & Cois, A. (2020). *240 Section A: universal health coverage index at district level box 1: Key measurement concepts for effective service coverage.*

NDOH. (2014). *South African national health normative standards framework for interoperability in eHealth government gazette version*, March 2014, pp.1–57.

O'Mahony, D. & Wright, G. (2014). Tablet computers for recording tuberculosis data at a community health centre in King Sabata Dalindyebo local municipality, Eastern Cape: A proof of concept report. *South African Family Practice*, 56(3), pp.186–189.

Odama, A. (2010). *Is there a link between the quality of clinical data ownership in the primary health care facilities of the Nyandeni Subdistrict?* Master's Thesis, M Sc Health Informatics, University of Winchester, Winchester.

Odama, A., Wright, G., Kabuya, C. & O'Mahony, D. (2014a). District of the Eastern Cape Province, South Africa: Project from data flow through coding to implementation using tablet computers. In EFMI Special Topic Conference, Budapest, Hungry, April, 27–29.

Odama, A., Wright, G., Kabuya, C., & O'Mahony, D. (2014b). Proof of concept using tablet computers to survey TB. In *Conference Proceedings for the 11th EFMI Special Topics, Studies in Health Technology and Informatics.* Budapest: IOS Press, p.129. https://doi.org/10.3233/978-1-61499-389-6-129

Osler, M. & Boulle, A. (2010). Three interlinked electronic registers (TIER.Net) project, (September), 1–9.

SAQA [online]. (2021). Available from: https://www.saqa.org.za/about-saqa (Accessed 15 May 2021).

Singh, J. A., Upshur, R., & Padayatchi, N. (2007). XDR-TB in South Africa: No time for denial or complacency. *PLoS Medicine*, 4(1), p.e50. https://doi.org/10.1371/journal.pmed.0040050.PMID: 17253901

Technical Guidance Publications [online]. (2020). Available at: https://www.who.int/emergencies/diseases/novel-coronavirus-2019/technical-guidance-publications (Accessed 28 May 2021).

UNAIDS. (2020). *AIDSinfo* [online]. *Aidsinfo.* Available at: http://aidsinfo.unaids.org

WHO. (2009). *WHO report...: Global tuberculosis control: epidemiology, strategy, financing.* Geneva, Switzerland: World Health Organization.

WHO. (2021a). *Nursing and midwifery indicators* [online]. The Global Health Observatory. Available at: https://www.who.int/data/gho/data/indicators/indicator-details/GHO/nursing-and-midwifery-personnel-(per-10–000-population) (Accessed 22 Aug 2021).

WHO. (2021b). *WHO. data statistics* [online]. Available at: http://www.who.int/hiv/data/en/ %0D%0A (Accessed 23 Feb 2021).

Wright, G. (2013). Evaluating the impact of technologies in clinical practice settings: An examination of research projects looking at nurses in rural clinics in the poorest area of South Africa. *Health Informatics New Zealand: Engaged*

Patients Rebalancing the Clinical Relationship. 2013 HINZ: Conference: Co-designing Health – Clinicians, Consumers and Executives Working together to Drive eHealth, Rotorua, New Zealand, December 4–5. Panel Presentation.

Wright, G. (2018). Some thoughts about health informatics in Africa. *European Journal for Biomedical Informatics*, 14(1), pp.13–15.

Wright, G. & Odama, A. (2012). Health data ownership and data quality: Clinics in the Nyandeni District, Eastern Cape, South Africa. *Engineering Management Research*, 1(2), pp.56–61.

Wright, G., Betts, H., Hernández Cáceres, J. L., Odama, A., O'Mahony, D., Yogeswaran, P., & Govere, F. (2014a). Issues and potential solutions when capturing health data in rural clinics in South Africa. *Revista Cubana de Informática Médica*, 6(1), pp.99–109.

Wright, G., Cillers, L., Van Niekerk, E., Seekoe, E., Cilliers, L., Van Niekerk, E., & Seekoe, E. (2017). The next stage of development of elearning at UFH in South Africa. In Proceedings of the International Conference on E-Learning, EL 2017: Part of the Multi Conference on Computer Science and Information Systems 2017.

Wright, G., O'Mahony, D., Kabuya, C., Betts, H. & Odama, A. (2014b). Nurses behaviour pre and post the implementation of data capture using tablet computers in a rural clinic in South Africa. *Studies in Health Technology and Informatics*, 210, pp.803–807.

Chapter 11

Teamwork and Informatics: Capturing the Work of Nurses as Team Members

Kristen K. Will and Gerri Lamb

Contents

Introduction

Healthcare is rediscovering the power of teams and teamwork. Faced with a pandemic, out-of-control costs and overwhelming evidence about health inequities in the US and globally, providers, administrators and policymakers alike are recognizing—once again—that teams harness expertise in ways that are impossible for individual providers to manage or duplicate. Research shows that high-performing teams, teams that optimize the contributions of

DOI: 10.4324/9781003054849-11

each member, deliver quality outcomes, reduce costs and serve as a safety net to preserve the quality of life and morale of their members.

Teamwork, and the call to teamwork, are not new for nurses. Most health services in the US and globally have been delivered by interprofessional teams for some time. While teamwork has been touted in certain specialty settings like hospice or rehabilitation, working in teams is the implicit norm across all settings from acute care to ambulatory care, long-term care and community. In each of these settings, nurses have and continue to hold critical roles as direct providers and as facilitators of core team processes, including communication and coordination. Their contributions in these latter roles are integral to improved outcomes including fewer hospitalizations and rehospitalizations, better control of chronic conditions and lower costs. It is not a coincidence that communication and coordination have been recognized by the Centers for Medicare and Medicaid Services as pivotal to quality outcomes (CMS, 2021). Nor should the call to reimburse teams rather than individual providers be seen as novel or surprising. Teams *are* the basic unit of healthcare today and high-performing teams deliver. This current focus on teams and recognition of their value in healthcare are long overdue.

What does this mean for nurses and team members? Why is the electronic health record important? Nurses have been and continue to be the backbone and glue of many, if not most, health teams. As billable providers, the work of advanced practice providers is discoverable although many of their distinctive contributions to quality outcomes and team performance are still not measured or tracked. In contrast, the roles and contributions of registered nurses as direct providers and team facilitators are mostly invisible in documentation and payment systems. Norma Lang, one of nursing's greatest champions for capturing nursing care in information systems, famously said that naming and measuring nursing's work are essential to improving it and being paid for it (Clark & Lang, 1992). While this is still true, we have a critical opportunity to capitalize on the synergy between available data and the growth of big data science to document, track, evaluate and improve the contributions of all team members, including nurses.

In this chapter, we highlight research findings that place teams in the center of healthcare delivery and provide examples of uses of the electronic health record to evaluate the impact of teams on healthcare outcomes. Further, we discuss the important role of the Electronic health records (EHR) in capturing the work of nurses and other team members in the context of individual and team roles. We offer exemplars of quality and research initiatives that leverage the EHR and big data science to improve our understanding of team performance and accurately evaluate the contributions of nurses and other team members. Finally, we make recommendations for optimizing the use of the EHR for the future of nursing and team practice, education and research.

Teamwork in Healthcare

There is a growing body of research demonstrating the impact of teamwork on the Quadruple Aim. Effective teamwork is associated with improved population health, lower costs and improved patient and provider experience. Specifically, teams caring for high-risk populations in the acute care setting have shown decreased readmission rates, decreased adverse events and length of stay during hospitalization and improved provider satisfaction (Boulding et al., 2011; Jha et al., 2008; Meterko et al., 2004; Wen & Schulman, 2014). In the ambulatory care setting, implementation of Patient-centered Medical Homes (PCMHs) that rely on interprofessional teamwork models has been studied in patient populations with many different chronic disease models, including diabetes mellitus, advanced heart failure and chronic kidney disease (Odum & Whaley-Connell, 2012). Extensive research has been conducted examining various patient outcomes within PCMHs for patients with multiple co-morbidities and high utilization rates of the healthcare system. These studies show significant improvement in outcomes for patients with complex, chronic disease related to improved disease management, decreased utilization of the healthcare system and lower healthcare costs when cared for by teams (Odum & Whaley-Connell, 2012; Reiss-Brennan et al., 2016). Further, teamwork is noted to be a lead recommendation to combat the opioid epidemic. The Centers for Disease Control (CDC) has listed interprofessional teams as a key intervention for effective treatment of populations suffering from substance abuse and dependence (Department of Health, Services, and for Disease Control, 2018).

Programs utilizing a team-based care approach also have shown reduced costs associated with lower use of expensive services, like hospitalizations and emergency room visits (Ahmed et al., 2012; Gade et al., 2008; Hung et al., 2013). Team-based care is hypothesized to reduce service use and costs by decreasing medical errors and redundancy in care (Mitchell et al., 2012; Reeves et al., 2013).

Healthcare teams also have been linked to improved patient experience through enhanced engagement and satisfaction. A systematic review by Will et al. (2019) explored the relationship between team-based care and patient satisfaction in the acute care setting and looked at the role of team composition and type of team intervention on this relationship. Both quasi-experimental and experimental studies were reviewed. Findings showed an overall positive relationship between team-based care and patient satisfaction. Additional studies indicate that teamwork may promote patient activation which is a component of patient engagement and linked with improved patient experience (Alexander et al., 2012; Shortell et al., 2017). Improving relationships and communication within the healthcare team also improve provider well-being and prevent burnout (Dai et al., 2020; Everett et al., 2018; Gittell et al., 2018).

The growing emphasis on team-based care has been accompanied by changes in the ways researchers and clinicians study teams and their outcomes. Many of the early studies conducted by social scientists were qualitative, based on extensive observation and ratings of team interactions (Schmitt et al., 1982). These studies laid a rich foundation for the movement into quantitative methods and the use of EHR data to evaluate team performance. The demand for more immediate demonstration of outcomes and greater generalizability across teams and settings has led to the current era of mixed methods research with greater use of quasi-experimental and experimental designs. Importantly, the conceptual underpinnings for team science continue to grow (Salas et al., 2009).

Through all these advances studying teams, which demonstrate the widespread positive effects of teamwork in healthcare, barriers to studying teams exist. Traditional ways of studying teams have been labor-intensive, lack replicability across diverse patient care settings and linkage to direct patient outcomes. This work utilized qualitative, observational data, which was laborious and lacked generalizability (Schmitt et al., 1982). More recent work studying teams uses quantitative, quasi-experimental and experimental research designs, but continues to lack direct connection to patient outcomes (Brandt et al., 2014; Reeves et al., 2013). Further, traditional methodologies of studying teams often focus on billable providers, using claims data as a source of quantitative data. This method omits important members of the team, such as nursing, hidden and lacking representation and attribution for their contribution to the team (Everett et al., 2019; Palmieri & Peterson, 2009). Going directly into the EHR to track nurse contributions and overall team performance will address many of these gaps.

Nurses and Teams

As noted earlier, teams are the basic unit of healthcare today. As the largest group of health professionals and the team member most likely to serve as the 'face' of the team to patients and families, the effectiveness of nursing care is closely tied to teamwork performance. Increasingly, all health professions are required to demonstrate interprofessional and collaborative competence (Health Professions Accreditors Collaborative, 2019). For nurses, this requirement is not new. However, the ever-increasing complexity of healthcare and the nurse's pivotal position at the intersections of all aspects of care delivery, necessitate they excel in teamwork performance, modeling and leadership.

The expectation and demand for teamwork competence are threaded through nursing scholarship and education. The theoretical foundations for nursing practice include core concepts like partnership, communication, and relationship building that are integral to effective team performance ((Reed, 2006). Interprofessional partnership is a major domain in nursing accreditation guidelines (AACN, 2021).

In practice, nurses play key roles in care coordination, communication and integration, that place them at the intersection of teams in every setting. Increasingly, these complex skills sets have been recognized as high-performance teamwork (Lamb and Newhouse, 2018). Research findings demonstrate these nursing roles and the interventions associated with them are highly correlated with quality and cost outcomes (Haas et al., 2014; Henson, 2010; Peikes et al., 2009).

The close association between professional nursing practice and their role as team connectors, facilitators, and leaders is one that needs to be better explicated for nurses to optimize their individual and collective impact. Being deeply embedded in team performance coupled with lack of ability to bill or be recognized in quality performance and billing systems for core functions like care coordination are recipes for invisibility and diminished impact. More effective use of the electronic health record to capture nursing care in the context of their vital team roles is a central part of solving this problem (AHRQ, 2017).

EHR and Teams

Electronic health records (EHRs) are a major source of longitudinal clinical information. They commonly incorporate or are connected to patient-generated information via patient portals and may be part of larger information networks across health settings and systems. Increasingly, they are being used as a source of quality data for public reporting and value-based quality metrics. The HITECH Act of 2009 encouraged healthcare providers to utilize electronic health records through offering reimbursement incentives, giving a significant boost to its use in quality and payment initiatives.

Documentation in the EHR is part of a longitudinal record of a patient's clinical care. Although there has been considerable movement toward a single integrated record for each patient, it is still time-consuming to track patient contacts and care across providers and settings. Time and motion studies of nurses in the hospital show that nurses spend considerable time documenting care and facilitating communication through the EHR (Hendrich et al., 2008). National and international surveys suggest that clinical documentation systems are a major source of dissatisfaction for nurses especially related to supporting their professional and teamwork responsibilities (Kutney-Lee et al., 2021; Topaz et al., 2017).

While not always optimized, EHRs have significant potential to support teamwork practice, improvement and research. Certain elements in the EHR, like care plans, provide real-time snapshots of team-based care. Documentation of transitions in care, such as transfer and discharge notes, are places in which team communication and handoffs are likely to be more visible.

Researchers are just beginning to turn to EHRs as a source of data to study healthcare teams. Two programs of study by Everett et al. (2018, 2019) and Pany et al. (2021) demonstrate its' considerable promise for studying teams and their impact on patient outcomes. Everett and colleagues used the EHR to explicate the relationship between team composition and patient outcomes associated with diabetes mellitus. Studying dyad teams and their impact on patients with diabetes mellitus, Everett et al. examined the various types of team combinations and their impact on diabetes outcome metrics. Pany et al. studying team-based care vs. solo physician or nonphysician provider care (NP or PA) and the impact on chronic disease management, found that team-based care was superior to solo practitioner care, regardless of the team composition and/or the solo practitioner discipline (Pany et al., 2021).

These early studies of the team using EHR data rely on billing data to identify team members and limited to team members able to bill directly for their services. Importantly, this research begins to capture the work of advanced practice providers on teams. It does not capture the work of registered nurses or other team members not in billing systems.

Building the potential to use EHR data to study teams is imperative to further understand their impact on clinical outcomes and the attribution of the team members. In this next section, we provide examples of strategies to accelerate the use of EHR to study team outcomes and to capture the work of nurses as members of teams. The first case study exemplar describes a theory-based approach to identifying a greater set of team members in primary care settings than is possible with billing data. This approach was part of a larger study to study and measure the relationship of primary care teams and a component of patient engagement, patient activation. It involved the implementation of a novel methodology of identifying primary care teams within raw EHR data, creating a 'team variable,' and measuring the impact on patient activation utilizing traditional statistical analysis and machine learning.

The second case study exemplar describes emerging opportunities to use the EHR to identify and improve nurse care coordination activities. It highlights actions needed to assure documentation in the EHR accurately represents the contributions nurse interventions make within teams to care coordination outcomes.

Case Study Exemplar 1: Finding the Team in the EHR

Discrete teams are not readily available in the EHR data and require a step-wise approach, underpinned by team theory and common definition(s) to find the teams in the EHR data. Working together, the dyad team of the clinician and data analyst first reviewed the data dictionary for discoverable data points that represented key constructs of teams and developed a process to organize the variables based on theory. A common definition for teams, *Interprofessional Team-Based Care*, and well-known team theories provide the constructs for identifying data dictionary variables and decision rules in the EHR (Table 11.1).

Once it was determined that big data relevant to teams existed and may be retrieved from the EHR, the dyad team moved into analysis. Advanced computational resources—available today as never before—allowed much more detailed exploration into team structure. While traditional statistical analysis (hierarchal regression, multilevel models, etc.) is effective for studying teams, researchers are turning to machine learning techniques to study this type of big data. Two different types of analysis were utilized to study primary care teams and their impact on patient activation, mixed level methods and machine learning. Recent research demonstrates that machine

Table 11.1   Aligning Theory, Definition, Data Variables and Decision Rules in HER

Theoretical	*Data Dictionary Variables*	*Decision Rule for EHR Data*
1. Patient-centered	• Patient demographic variables and associated outcome variable(s) • Provider type	• Create data table of desired patient population • Identify all provider types associated with patient population
2. Intentionally created	• Encounter location (billable and non-billable)—ambulatory care • Encounter type (primary care) • Provider types and primary care medical home location	• Associate all provider types with the patient population associated with primary care visits only • Limit provider types to those associated with patient' primary care medical home location
3. Interprofessional	• Provider type (RN, Physician, NP, PA, MA, etc.)	• Two or more different healthcare disciplines
4. Shared goals	• Provider type (primary care medical home) and Encounter types associated with DM2 diagnosis (ICD codes)	• Connect providers based on common patient diagnosis(es) such as Diabetes Mellitus

learning may replicate validity and reliability similar to randomized-controlled trials (Mehta & Devarakonda, 2018).

Case Study Exemplar 2: Nurse Care Coordination in the EHR

Capturing care coordination interventions in the EHR and attributing them to various team members is challenging. Care coordination incorporates multiple elements including assessment of patient risk and social determinants of health, development of an integrated plan of care, and communication among multiple providers and services. The process requires assessment, monitoring and tracking over time and exquisite attention to timing and sequencing of care and services. In addition, payment for care coordination is highly prescribed and determined by algorithms around patient complexity and other variables (CMS, 2019).

Numerous stakeholders have grappled with defining and measuring care coordination. The nursing community has emphasized the importance of these efforts to achieve national quality goals and health equity and for nurses to be recognized and reimbursed for care coordination interventions (Lamb et al., 2015; National Academies of Sciences, Engineering and Medicine, 2021). Increasingly, the EHR is being looked to as a source of real-time data to document, evaluate and improve care coordination. We can anticipate that within a few years, greater numbers of EHR-based measures of care coordination will be used for public reporting and incentives associated with value-based care.

As we move toward greater reliance on the EHR to document the delivery and quality of team-based interventions, like care coordination, and their outcomes, all health professionals who contribute to these outcomes will need to be able to point to where and how their interventions are documented. While narrative descriptions may be easier to excerpt and translate into quality metrics in the future, quality reporting will likely remain based on quantitative formats, such as the percent of patients discharged from the hospital with a plan of care or follow-up visit with their primary care provider.

Nurses can take several steps to prepare to maximize the opportunity to assure their care coordination activities are discoverable in the EHR and able to be distinguished within team-based care. Immediate actions include:

■ Have consensus definitions of major nurse care coordination prepared and available to organizations testing and vetting care coordination measures for use in the EHR.
■ Identify locations for documentation of care coordination interventions in EHR, such as the integrated plan of care and use them consistently.
■ Examine how nurse care coordination interventions are documented in preparation for their quantification and identify opportunities to translate the narrative into numbers.
■ Work with measure developers on ways to distinguish team inputs within care coordination documentation and measurement.

Recommendations for Practice, Education and Research

The EHR offers significant opportunities to use the EHR to study teams and advance nursing practice, education and research. Specific actions that will assist nurses in realizing these goals include:

1. Prepare for reimbursement changes

Several reports, including the Future of Nursing 2020-2030, recommend changes in payment to recognize the contributions of nurses to healthcare outcomes (National Academy of Medicine, 2021). We can anticipate that these changes will be accompanied by new requirements for documentation and performance measures. In preparation, nurses in all settings need to explore the potential of their current EHRs to accommodate new data and tools that will capture their work. It will be particularly important to align data capture with quality measures used for organizational accreditation and value-based reporting.

2. Develop models for team attribution

Data analysis models that parse quality outcomes by team member contributions are in the earliest stages of development. It will be important for nurses to join committees designing and testing these models to provide input about the competencies and time required for the interventions under consideration. Formulas for attributing the work of each team member to targeted quality and cost outcomes will require close scrutiny and testing.

These models are likely to be controversial. Resolving issues related to accurate and equitable team-based payment will require considerable dialogue and negotiation among the health professions and policymakers.

3. Address EHR usability

Recent studies have shown a significant correlation between EHR usability and adverse nurse and patient outcomes (Kutney-Lee et al., 2021; Topaz et al., 2017). Issues related to slow access to patient data, concerns about accuracy, and difficulty sharing information need to be resolved to optimize the use of the EHR to support teamwork.

4. Use EHR to full capacity

Much of the literature indicates that EHR platforms are not used to full capacity (Rudin et al., 2020). Nurses and other providers often rely on them solely for basic functions available in standard packages. They may not be aware of additional functionality to support clinical processes or told that changes are cost-prohibitive. Rather than be put off by the barriers, nurses and their team members need to be encouraged to work with HIT staff and administrators on creative and less costly solutions to make EHRs work for the healthcare team and their goals improving quality processes and outcomes.

5. Leverage current EHR data to study and improve teamwork

As EHR platforms evolve, more data points will be available and easier to mine. Some EHR platforms have begun to identify 'treatment teams' as a discoverable data variable in data dictionary. This variable is currently created by provider types 'opting in' to the team and thus, remains user-dependent. In time, we can anticipate that EHR platforms will become more sophisticated to connect provider types automatically with patient populations to create the treatment team and drive attribution and payment.

Increased use of machine learning techniques to analyze big data, such as described in the case study exemplar illustrated above, will accelerate efficient access and use of more EHR data for practice and research. This will have a considerable impact on our ability to match team structures and processes to the needs of different populations. Nurse researchers will play an important role in guiding decisions about data to include in models used to connect team processes and outcomes. The Interprofessional Education Core Data Set supported by the National Center for Interprofessional Practice and Education, is an example of a readily available data set which nurse researchers can utilize to study teams and their outcomes (Delaney et al., 2020). Including EHR data, the IPE Core Data Set includes six components: critical IPE events, Interprofessional Collaborative Competencies Attainment Survey (ICCAS), interprofessional clinical learning environment, interprofessional education learning environment, teamness measurements (ACE-15), and outcomes (quadruple aim).

Conclusion

Healthcare teams are more imperative than ever for delivery of high quality, patient-centered care. With the exponential growth of big data and further refinement of interoperability across EHR platforms, the study and measure of teams within EHR data has immense potential. Opportunities include identification of team member attribution for all members of the healthcare team, further study of real-life clinical outcomes in relationship to healthcare teams, and implication for policy and reimbursement of teamwork. The use of EHR data includes a systematic process of data mining, data analytics and interpretation, potentiated through a collaboration between data scientists, informaticists and clinicians. This chapter proposes a process to systematically engage in team research using the EHR, including areas of nursing practice to focus on, establishing a foundation for mining EHR data that will build science and improve practice across the continuum for healthcare teams.

References

Agency for Healthcare Research and Quality (AHRQ). (2017). *About the national quality strategy*. Rockville, MD: Agency for Healthcare Research and Quality. Retrieved from http://www.ahrq.gov/workingforquality/about/index.html.

Ahmed, N., Taylor, K., McDaniel, Y., & Dyer, C. B. (2012). The role of an acute care for the elderly unit in achieving hospital quality indicators while caring for frail hospitalized elders. *Population Health Management*, 15(4), pp.236–240. https://doi.org/10.1089/pop.2011.0055

Alexander, J. A., Hearld, L. R., Mittler, J. N., & Harvey, J. (2012). Patient-physician role relationships and patient activation among individuals with chronic illness. *Health Services Research*, 47(3 PART 1), pp.1201–1223. https://doi.org/10.1111/j.1475-6773.2011.01354.x

American Association of Colleges of Nursing (AACN). (2021). *Core competencies for professional nursing education*. Available at: www.aacnnursing.org (Accessed December 27, 2021).

Boulding, W., Glickman, S. W., Manary, M. P., Schulman, K. A., & Staelin, R. (2011). Relationship between patient satisfaction with inpatient care. *The American Journal of Managed Care*, 17(1), pp.41–48.

Brandt, B., Lutfiyya, M. N., King, J. A., & Chioreso, C. (2014). A scoping review of interprofessional collaborative practice and education using the lens of the Triple Aim. *Journal of Interprofessional Care*, 28(5), pp.393–399. https://doi.org/10.3109/13561820.2014.906391

Centers for Medicare and Medicaid Services (CMS) Meaningful Measures Hub. (2021). *Meaningful Measures Hub | CMS*. Available at: www.cms.gov (Accessed December 27, 2021).

Centers for Medicare and Medicaid Services (CMS) Medicare Learning Network. (2019). *Chronic care management services*. Retrieved from http://cms.gov/outreach-and-education/medicare-learning-network-mln/mlnproducts/downloads/chroniccaremanagement

Clark, J., & Lang, L., (1992). Nursing's next advance: An internal classification for nursing practice. *International Nursing Review*, 39(4), pp.109–111.

Dai, M., Willard-Grace, R., Knox, M., Larson, S. A., Magill, M. K., Grumbach, K., & Peterson, L. E. (2020). Team configurations, efficiency, and family physician burnout. *Journal of the American Board of Family Medicine*, 33(3), pp.368–377. https://doi.org/10.3122/jabfm.2020.03.190336

Delaney, C. W., AbuSalah, A., Yeazel, M., Stumpf Kertz, J., Pejsa, L., & Brandt, B. F. (2020 August). National center for interprofessional practice and education IPE core data set and information exchange for knowledge generation. *Journal of Interprofessional Care*, 18, pp.1–13. https://doi.org/10.1080/13561820.2020. 1798897. Epub ahead of print. PMID: 32811224.

Department of Health, U., Services, H., & for Disease Control, C. (2018). *Implementing the CDC guideline for prescribing opioids for chronic pain.* Retrieved from https://www.cdc.gov/drugoverdose/pdf/prescribing/CDC-DUIP-QualityImprovementAndCareCoordination-508.pdf

Everett, C. M., Morgan, P., Smith, V. A., Woolson, S., Edelman, D., Hendrix, C. C., Berkowitz, T., White, B., & Jackson, G. L. (2018). Interpersonal continuity of primary care of veterans with diabetes: A cohort study using electronic health record data. *BMC Family Practice*, 19(1), pp.1–11. https://doi.org/10.1186/s128 75-018-0823-5

Everett, C. M., Morgan, P., Smith, V. A., Woolson, S., Edelman, D., Hendrix, C. C., Berkowitz, T., White, B., & Jackson, G. L. (2019). Primary care provider type: Are there differences in patients' intermediate diabetes outcomes? *JAAPA : Official Journal of the American Academy of Physician Assistants*, 32(6), pp.36–42. https://doi.org/10.1097/01.JAA.0000558239.06875.0b

Gade, G., Venohr, I., Conner, D., McGrady, K., Beane, J., Richardson, R. H., Williams, M. P., Liberson, M., Blum, M., & Penna, R. D. (2008). Impact of an inpatient palliative care team: A randomized controlled trial. *Journal of Palliative Medicine*, *11*(2), pp.180–190. https://doi.org/10.1089/jpm.2007.0055

Gittell, J. H., Logan, C., Cronenwett, J., Foster, T. C., Freeman, R., Godfrey, M., & Vidal, D. C. (2018). Impact of relational coordination on staff and patient outcomes in outpatient surgical clinics. *Health Care Management Review*, 1. https://doi.org/10.1097/HMR.0000000000000192

Haas, S. A., Swan, B. A., & Haynes, T. S., eds. (2014). *Care coordination and transition management core curriculum*. Pittman, NJ: American Academy of Ambulatory Care Nursing.

Health Professions Accreditors Collaborative. (2019). Guidance on developing quality interprofessional education for the health professions. Chicago, IL: Health Professions Accreditors Collaborative. Retrieved from https://healthprofessio nsaccreditors.org/wp-content/uploads/2019/02/HPACGuidance02-01-19.pdf

Hendrich, A., Chow, M. P., Skierczynski, B. A., & Lu, Z. (2008). A 36-hospital time and motion study: How do medical surgical nurses spend their time. *The Permanente Journal*, 12(3), pp.25–34.

Henson, A. (2010). Practitioner application: A method for defining value in healthcare using cancer care as a model. *Journal of Healthcare Management*, 55(6), pp.411–412. https://doi.org/10.1097/00115514-201011000-00007

Hung, W. W., Ross, J. S., Farber, J., & Siu, A. L. (2013). Evaluation of the mobile acute care of the elderly (MACE) service. *JAMA Internal Medicine*, 173(11), pp.990–996. https://doi.org/10.1001/jamainternmed.2013.478

Jha, A. K., Orav, E. J., Zheng, J., & Epstein, A. M. (2008). Patients' perception of hospital care in the United States. *New England Journal of Medicine*, 359(18), pp.1921–1931. https://doi.org/10.1056/NEJMsa0804116

Kutney-Lee, A., Carthon, M. B., Sloane, D. M., Bowles, K. H., McHugh, M. D., & Aiken, L. H. (2021). Electronic health record usability: Associations with nurse and patient outcomes in hospitals. *Medical Care*, 2021. https://doi:10.1097/MLR.625-631, 0000000000001536

Lamb, G., & Newhouse, R. (2018). *Care coordination: A blueprint for action for RNs*. Silver Spring, MD: American Nurses Association.

Lamb, G., Newhouse, R., Beverly, C., Toney, D. A., Cropley, S., Weaver, C. A., Kurtzman, E., Zazworsky, D., Rantz, M., Zierler, B. & Naylor, M. (2015). Policy agenda for nurse-led care coordination. *Nursing Outlook*, 63(4), pp.521–530. https://doi.org/10.1016/j.outlook.2015.06.003

Mehta, N., & Devarakonda, M. V. (2018). Machine learning, natural language programming, and electronic health records: The next step in the artificial intelligence journey? *Journal of Allergy and Clinical Immunology*, 141(6), pp.2019-2021.e1. https://doi.org/10.1016/j.jaci.2018.02.025

Meterko, M., Mohr, D. C., & Young, G. J. (2004). Teamwork culture and patient satisfaction in hospitals. *Medical Care*, 42(5), pp.492–498. https://doi.org/10.1097/01.mlr.0000124389.58422.b2

Mitchell, P., Wynia, M., Golden, R., Mcnellis, B., Okun, S., Webb, C. E., Rohrbach V, & Von Kohorn, I. (2012). *Core principles & values of effective team-based health care*. Retrieved from www.iom.edu/tbc.

National Academy of Medicine. (2021). *Future of nursing 2020–2030: Charting a path to achieve health equity*. Retrieved from https://nam.edu/publications/the-future-of-nursing-2020-2030/?gclid=CjwKCAjw7J6EBhBDEiwA5UUM2ij1cfJDn6Occcrir4jdywBlA9u_xA6Zmuua2gaCy2n9srbULknp3xoCquQQAvD_BwE

Odum, L., & Whaley-Connell, A. (2012). The role of team-based care involving pharmacists to improve cardiovascular and renal outcomes. *Cardiorenal Medicine*, 2(4), pp.243–250. https://doi.org/10.1159/000341725

Palmieri, P. A., & Peterson, L. T. (2009). Attribution theory and healthcare culture: Translational management science contributes a framework to identify the etiology of punitive clinical environments. *Advances in Health Care Management*, 8, pp.81–111. https://doi.org/10.1108/S1474-8231(2009)0000008008

Pany, M. J., Chen, L., Sheridan, B., & Huckman, R. S. (2021). Provider teams outperform solo providers in managing chronic diseases and could improve the value of care. *Health Affairs*, 40(3), pp.435–444. https://doi.org/10.1377/hlthaff.2020.01580

Peikes D, Chen A, Schore J, & Brown, R. (n.d.). Effects of care coordination on hospitalization,quality of care, and health care expenditures among medicare beneficiaries: 15 Randomized Trials. *JAMA*, 301(6), pp.603–618. doi:10.1001/jama.2009.126

Reed, P. G. (2006). Commentary on neomoderism and evidence-based nursing: Implications for the production of nursing knowledge. *Nursing Outlook*, 54, pp.36–38.

Reeves, S., Perrier, L., Freeth, D., & Zwarenstein, M. (2013). Interprofessional education: Effects on professional practice and healthcare outcomes (update) (review). *Cochrane Database of Systematic Reviews*, 3. https://doi.org/10.4028/www.scientific.net/AMR.542-543.271

Reiss-Brennan, B., Brunisholz, K. D., Dredge, C., Briot, P., Grazier, K., Wilcox, A., Savitz, L., & James, B. (2016). Association of integrated team-based care with health care quality, utilization, and cost. *JAMA: Journal of the American Medical Association*, 316(8), pp.826–834. https://doi.org/10.1001/jama.2016.11232

Rudin, R. S., Fischer, S. H., Damberg, C. L., Shi, Y., Shekelle, P. G., Xenakis, L., Khodyakov, D., & Ridgely, M. S. (2020, December). Optimizing health IT to improve health system performance: A work in progress. *Healthcare*, 8(4), p.100483. Elsevier.

Salas, E., Almeida, S. A., Salisbury, M., King, H., Lazzara, E. H., Lyons, R., Wilson, K. A., Almeida, P. A., & McQuillan, R. (2009). What are the critical success factors for team training in health care? *The Joint Commission Journal on Quality and Patient Safety*, 35(8), pp.398–405.

Schmitt, M., Watson, N., Feiger, S., & Williams, T. (1982). Conceptualizing and measuring outcomes of interdisciplinary team care for a group of long-term chronically ill, institutionalized patients. In Interdisciplinary Health Care: Proceedings of the Third Annual Interdisciplinary Team Care Conference, pp.169–182.

Shortell, S. M., Poon, B. Y., Ramsay, P. P., Rodriguez, H. P., Ivey, S. L., Huber, T., Rich, J., & Summerfelt, T. (2017). A multilevel analysis of patient engagement and patient-reported outcomes in primary care practices of accountable care organizations. *Journal of General Internal Medicine*, 32(6), pp.640–647. https://doi.org/10.1007/s11606-016-3980-z

Topaz, M., Ronquillo, C., Peltonen, L., Pruinelli, L., Sarmiento, R. F., Badger, M. K., Ali, S., Lewis, A., Georgsson, M., Jeon, E., Tayaben, J. L., Kuo, C. H., Islam, T., Sommer, J., Jung, H., Eler, G. J., Alhuwail, D., & Lee, Y. L. (2017). Nurse informaticians report low satisfaction and multi-level concerns with electronic health records: Results from an international survey. In AMIA Annual Symposium Proceedings, Washington, DC, pp.2016–2025.

Wen, J., & Schulman, K. A. (2014). Can team-based care improve patient satisfaction? A systematic review of randomized controlled trials. *PLoS ONE*, 9(7), pp.1–9. https://doi.org/10.1371/journal.pone.0100603

Will, K. K., Johnson, M. L., & Lamb, G. (2019). Team-based care and patient satisfaction in the hospital setting: A systematic review. *Journal of Patient-centered Research and Reviews*, 6(2), p.158.

Index